A gift for

February
Light

Also by Heather Trexler Remoff

Sexual Choice

February Light

Light

A Love Letter to the Seasons
During a Year of Cancer and Recovery

Heather Trexler Remoff

St. Martin's Press ❧ New York

Design by Nancy Resnick

Grateful acknowledgment is given for permission to reprint lines from "Nothing Gold Can Stay" from *The Poetry of Robert Frost,* edited by Edward Connery Lathem. Copyright 1951 by Robert Frost. Copyright 1923, © 1969 by Henry Holt & Co., Inc. Reprinted by permission of Henry Holt & Co., Inc.

Library of Congress Cataloging-in-Publication Data

Remoff, Heather Trexler.
    February light :   a love letter to the seasons during a year of cancer and recovery / Heather Trexler Remoff.
        p.   cm.
    ISBN 0-312-16839-X
    1. Remoff, Heather Trexler—Health.   2. Ovaries—Cancer—
Patients—Pennsylvania—Biography.   I. Title.
RC280.08.R46   1997
362.1'9699465'0092—dc21
    [B]   97-16245
                                                                        CIP

First Edition: September 1997

10   9   8   7   6   5   4   3   2   1

*To the doctors and staff in the Oncology Department
at Geisinger Medical Center in Danville
and to Ann Marie Wishard and the crew at Sweet Annie Herbs
in Centre Hall*

Acknowledgments

A great number of people play a part in the making of a book. This particular volume started not as an idea but as an emotion: gratitude. My family and friends have always given my life meaning. Therefore many of them are players in this book, and I hope that they will read my thanks in the stories I tell. Others, equally important, didn't make it into these pages and will inadvertently be left out of the abbreviated list that follows. So, a book that started with gratitude ends with apology. It is not possible to include the names of all those whose simple presence in the world is part of that world's hold on me.

Having said that, I thank Nonie Baker, Louisa Bushey, George Collins, Dick and Kathleen Deasy, Marge and Dave Finke, Mel and Gordon Fletcher-Howell, Frank and Vera Foulke, Kim Fried, Charlie and Amy Gardner, Laurie Gerlach, Donna and Jerry Gilbert, Edie Gordon, Jean Gould, Gib Halverson, Gary Hennen, Don and Donna Iarkowski, Abby and Harriet Jacobson, James Lane, Dave and Diane Lenhart, Stu and Nina Levitt, Lucy and Michael Muth, Lisa Pline, Harrell and Ivory Roberts, Sarah Shaffer, Bea Sims, Bob and Susan Zelten, and, always, Paul Heyer.

In addition to the friends and family who shape my world, there are the professionals who shape a book. My agent, Kay Kidde, and her associate, Laura Langlie, have been enthusiastic, supportive, and hard working. Kay's sense that my book belonged at St. Martin's has been confirmed by the happy experience this venture has been. Kelley Ragland, my editor at St. Martin's, has kept me informed and involved. Kelley understands the power of positive feedback. Her letters are guaranteed to keep any writer writing.

Finally, I owe so very much to the enchanted town of Osprey Lakes. Its name has been changed, as have the names of some of its residents. But the town is real. Its mountaintop location, its woods and lake, its air and light, and its people have all been central to my healing.

I was born in 1938. I still remember a fight, or at least one line from a fight, I had with my sister forty-five years ago. It's funny how over time small things can achieve a symbolic importance that so far outweighs any significance one would ascribe to them at the moment. In one angry sentence Sandy ended the quarrel and summed up my personality: "The trouble with you," she told me, "is that whatever you get, you pretend that's what you want."

Chapter 1

May

Osprey Lakes is one thing I didn't have to pretend to want. From the first time my husband, Gene, and I set foot in the place, it wasn't a matter of wanting or not wanting, it was a question of logistics. We knew we were home. What started as a vacation ended as a love affair. And as with all true love affairs, we enjoy reminiscing over each little twist of fate that brought us here. The importance of those events is recognized only in hindsight. However, when something feels this right, the recounting doesn't elicit panic as in "What if you hadn't had a rotten day?" or "What if we hadn't had a dog?" but only serves to reinforce the inevitability of the outcome. This was meant to happen, every piece of it.

Osprey Lakes is a tiny Victorian resort. It sits on top of a mountain in north-central Pennsylvania. Proudly billed as "the town that time forgot," the village, with a year-round population of 123, consists of a small cluster of shops and houses. The emotional center of Osprey Lakes is a mile-long, crystal-clear natural lake. That first weekend here, I scribbled a postcard to a friend: "I feel as if every positive energy force in the world intersects directly over the lake." That was before I'd heard any of the lore claiming that various Indian tribes once met on the shores and conducted their annual purification rites in its waters. That was before I had read the old turn-of-the-century brochures describing waters magically high in borax, a tonic to body and spirit and responsible for the radiant complexions of those who swam here.

Would the claims stand up to historical and scientific scrutiny? I don't care. They match the personal truth I experience in these mountains. The path from center-city Philadelphia to permanent residence in Sullivan County, where one must drive forty-five minutes to find a grocery store that consistently stocks lettuce other than iceberg, is surely of less interest to the reader than it is to Gene and me. We did it in stages, each one flowing out of the one before with the inevitability of fate.

May is the month that marks the beginning of our years as homeowners in Osprey Lakes. Abandoning all regard for sound financial management and a secure old age, we bought one of the Victorian cottages. I've said this was a love affair, and true to the nature of such adventures, all our decisions were romantic rather than practical. These "cottages" are cottage in name only. Our home, Fitch Cottage, was built around 1883 and has seven bedrooms if one fails to count the four basement-level rooms where the servants slept. That was in 1883. In 1989 I liked to remind myself that I was the only "servant." However, in my case, the mistress was the house, and my labors were performed for love, not money.

The first time we saw the house, we were looking for a summer rental. It was late winter. We walked through mud and the dull remains of ice to get to the front door. The Realtor turned the key, and as I stepped over the threshold, I heard my own voice say something totally out of keeping with my normally frugal character: "I don't want to rent it. I want to buy it." The rugs were rolled up. The furniture was covered with sheets. Semidehydrated dead mice and mothballs dotted the floor. But from that moment on, the house claimed me. Gene and I ended up buying the cottage, but we have never owned it. Somehow Fitch made that clear to us from the first. We are here as resident caretakers, temporary employees, necessarily temporary, for the house predated our fleeting existence on this earth and will continue to capture and charm long after we are gone.

Victorians, at least Victorians with enough money to build a house intended for occupancy only two or three months of the year, understood leisure. A wide porch wraps around Fitch, climaxing in a circular sitting area filled with wicker furniture that may have been there since the house was built. Most of the old cottages in Osprey Lakes are sold furnished. Since they are second homes, and large ones at that, sellers generally are content to leave the furniture with the property. I think there is more to it than that. These houses are filled with ghosts of the past. Left cold and empty nine months of the year, they develop proprietary airs that only the extremely strong-willed can successfully challenge. Fitch Cottage came fully furnished. She understood what was rightfully hers. That was part of her charm.

But there is more to her charm than the furniture. Her interior walls are floor-to-ceiling wood that glows with the patina of over one hundred years. The first floor is not really separated into rooms in the conventional sense, but is an expanse of space defined by columns and arches, great arcades that mark the divide between dining, living, reading, and entry areas. There is a wide, open staircase with a window seat at the landing. The windows themselves are edged with small, diamond-shaped panes. Only when the sun is at a low morning or evening angle does light shine into the center of the first floor, for this is a house designed to be cool. And the design is so successful that, even in the summer months, there are days when the big brick fireplace in the living room is called into action to take the edge off an evening chill.

All of the old cottages here have fireplaces. Since the cottages were not intended for anything but summer use, they do not have central heat. Everyone in Osprey Lakes told us that it would be impossible to winterize Fitch, and, of course, everyone was right, but we did it anyway. Everyone told us we couldn't live in this house year-round, and, of course, everyone was right, but we do it anyway. Without regret. Until a person has been owned by a house in the way we are owned by this one, it is impossible to make one understand the lengths to which we will go to accommodate her.

Although we officially took ownership of Fitch in January, it was not simply lack of heat that kept us from moving in until May. It was also lack of water. The town water supply in Osprey Lakes is a seasonal system. It uses water from the lake; the ancient aqueducts, like so much else in this town, were designed with summer in mind. The pipes are close enough to the surface that they would freeze during our bitterly cold winters. Those who live here year-round all have private wells. However, it wasn't entirely a belief that the town ceased to exist, Brigadoon-fashion, between the months of September and May that kept the water pipes close to the surface. Our mountaintop is largely rock. Even planting daffodil bulbs is a challenge. No shovel goes very deep without becoming acquainted with the hard facts of our existence.

May 15 is the official date for turning on the water. We have a plumbing dynasty in our town. As soon as the frost is reliably out of the ground, one can see the Housts, our third-generation family of plumbers, moving soundlessly through the backyards. Every now and then, they stoop down and appear to reach directly into the earth. The hand is lost to view, but the arm twists, turning on the valves hidden beneath rocks, opening the water lines. They could hold us all hostage to their expertise if they wished. To my knowledge, there is no map detailing the location of these stopcocks. The legends are internal, passed from grandfather on down. It is a true ritual of spring, the start of the summer season. However, because this month can be a very cool one, few summer people are here to mark the occasion with appropriate fanfare.

When we bought the house, Gene was still working in Philadelphia. We intended to summer here until he was ready for retirement some eight or ten years down the road. Fitch had other ideas. The day after we closed the sale, Gene said, "This would be a perfect place for you to write." It didn't take much more persuasion than that. I moved in five months later. We sold our house in Philadelphia. Gene rented a small apartment close to his office and began a weekend commute that has no doubt introduced its own bit of unreliability into census tract data. When the census taker asked me how long it took my husband to get to work, I replied, "Monday morning, it's three and a half hours. Tuesday, it's five minutes."

May in Osprey Lakes is magical. The beginning of the month can still pretend to winter. In fact, after our first weekend that first May, Gene headed back to the city on Sunday night, leaving me alone in a big, old, unfamiliar house in a deserted town. Ours was the only home on the main thoroughfare with year-round occupancy. Our bedroom is on the third floor. Sometime in the night, the temperature began a steady drop. The furnace, cast-iron radiators, and miles of copper pipe that would eventually make us at least look like a winterized home had not yet been installed. The wind rattled the closed windows, sending the sheer curtains billowing about like tethered spirits. The old house shook to the extent that I could feel the bed tremble. I thought I heard footsteps on the stairs, and I *know* I heard doors banging. Although bed linens came with the house, there were no heavy blankets, and I shivered through the night. Curled in a tight, body-heat-conserving ball, I would have bargained with all those door-slamming spooks for a pair of wool socks, a hat to pull down over my ears. By morning it was strangely quiet. Had the world fallen away? Were this bedroom and I all that remained, the only things that had not been carried off? I crept over to the window and saw a universe very much there but completely transformed by eight inches of snow.

By the end of the month, the hybrid rhododendrons are heavy with bloom. A scattering of spring bulbs marks those yards with permanent residents. The Laurel Path, which circles the lake, is lined not only with laurel but with buttercups, forget-me-nots, painted trillium. All the old lawns and the woods and the cracks in the sidewalks are alive with violets. It was through violets that I first got to know Willis.

Willis came with our house. "There's a man who does the grass," the previous owners told us. "He'll just show up when it needs cutting. You never have to call him. He'll bring your bill around at the end of the summer."

I start every day with a five-mile run. One morning when I got back, our lawn was perfectly mowed, but although I could hear the soft purring of a distant lawn mower, there was no sign of the mysterious Willis. Curious, I began to ask about him around town and soon had a whole collection of Willis legends before I'd ever met the man.

"Oh, that Willis, he'll only mow in a straight line," said one woman who for two years running had lost a curving flower border to the efficiency of Willis's riding mower. Nonetheless, she wouldn't dream of having anyone else do her lawns. As I learned that October when Willis came with our tally for his summer's work, his price is definitely right, but there is more to him than that. No one talks about Willis very long without mentioning his absolute honesty, his absolute reliability.

"He's been doing the lawns ever since I can remember," a fellow picking up his mail in the post office volunteered. "How old a man is he?" I wanted to know. My respondent laughed. "I asked him that once. He told me, 'Not ninety,' but he didn't say which side of ninety he fell on."

"Oh, that Willis. One summer we were going to fly to France for a few weeks," another woman informed me. "I thought I'd better tell him we were going and that he should just keep on with the grass till we got back. I asked him if he wanted me to pay him in advance. 'Oh, no,' he told me. 'I never take my pay before October.' " The woman continued her tale, "I forgot the whole incident, but a few days later Willis was back. 'Did you tell me you were going to *fly* to France?' When I nodded my confirmation, he said, 'Well, in that case, maybe you *had* better pay me in advance.' I want to tell you, it took some of the fun out of the vacation. I thought maybe Willis knew something we did not."

Willis has been out of the area only once in his "not ninety" years. He traveled to Philadelphia to visit a married daughter. "I didn't like it," he told me. "So I've stayed to home ever since."

"Don't ever try to negotiate with Willis," a local man well-grounded in the ins and outs of Osprey Lakes once advised me. "You can count it as a win if you end up in the same place where you started. At the end of an encounter with Willis, most folks find themselves set back a few paces. There used to be a kind of crazy lady came up here summers. You know, she always thought somebody was trying to break into her house in the middle of the night. I'd have to go on over and check it out. Never was anybody there. Well, one day she says to me, 'You know that big maple in my back yard?' Now, of course, I knew the tree. 'Well,' she says, 'do you suppose you could cut that tree down for me?' Now, of course, I could, but I didn't know why anybody would want to, but she wanted it done, and so I cut it down. Then she says to me, 'Do you suppose you could pull out that stump and fill it in with topsoil and plant a little grass?' Now, of course, I could, and so I did, and pretty soon she just had a solid piece of lawn back there. She called me over when Willis came to mow, think she wanted some kind of proof of all we'd done. She motioned Willis off his mower and pointed to the new patch of lawn. 'I had that tree cut down, Willis. My lawn is easier to mow now that you don't have to go around the tree. Since it's easier to do my lawn, you should charge me less money.' Well, Willis, he stood back and studied the situation for a few minutes. Then he said, 'The way I figure it is, there's more lawn to mow now, and I oughta charge you *more.*' And then he turned and got back on his tractor and just kept on with his mowing."

As I said, I met Willis over violets, and it was my first and last attempt to negotiate with him. The back lawn of our house slopes down to the lake. Ingrid and Craig, my grown children, tease me that I must have been a servant in Fitch cottage in a former life. The former-life business would certainly explain my instant affinity for the place, but what Ing and Craig especially have in mind is my total comfort in the basement level. I have set up my office in one of the old servants' bedrooms, and there I spend my days, dreaming and writing and gazing out at the lake. Because our house is built on a hill, even the lake side of the basement has large, above-ground windows, and I draw a writer's comfort from all that water. "You have a twelve-room house to write in," Ingrid tells me. "Why lock yourself in the basement?" She is teasing a bit. Being a writer herself, she understands the need to hide away somewhere from noise and other people. But what she doesn't understand— and I promise this is leading back to Willis—is why I so adore doing the laundry.

This house has a clothesline, a real clothesline. You know, the old-fashioned kind that has pulleys on either end. Oh, what a clothesline! In a house filled with wonderful features, this clothesline can make my soul sing. One pulley is anchored high on the basement back porch. The other is close to the sky in a tall black-locust tree. The bed linens that came with this house are all 100 percent cotton, and neatly chain-stitched in blue embroidery thread in the corner of each sheet is the name of one of the grand old Victorian hotels that was torn down years before our arrival on the mountain. The Lakeside. The sheets are white, of course. I love laundering them. That clothesline will hold the sheets from seven beds, not even a pole needed to prop them up away from the raspberry canes that border the yard. They just hang up there, waving high between the porch and the locust tree. The sun bleaches the sheets so white that, when they are on the line, it is impossible to look straight at them without squinting.

It was while I was hanging one of my many loads of glorious laundry, in preparation for a Memorial Day weekend brimming with houseguests, that I met Willis. I heard his mower before I saw him. Listening to it move across the neighboring lawns, growing ever closer to our own, I mentally calculated the height of my sheets and was certain that Willis's mower would fit easily under them. Not that it mattered this time. I didn't want Willis to cut the lawn. I wanted him to wait a week. The violets were the reason. The bottom third of our lawn was solid purple with violets. Since that first year, I have come to count on their absolutely reliable display just in time for the holiday. The entire lawn is laced through with violets, but the concentration is so great at the lower end that they form a dense mass of vibrant color. I wanted my houseguests to see the violets. There was no way I was going to let Willis cut them.

He parked his mower between our lawn and the neighbor's. I suppose I have to confess to loving Willis from the first moment I laid eyes on him, though of course all the stories had set me up. He is not a tall man. Years spent in the woods felling trees, and not always getting quickly enough out of the way of their crashing parts, have left their mark on Willis. He leans slightly forward from the waist. Arthritis has settled in his knees and hands and twisted him ever so slightly, like a towel ready to be rung out just when the housewife was interrupted and called off by some other task. The best part of Willis is his face. What makes a face honest? A direct gaze, of course, but that can be assumed. Willis's eyes are pale, pale blue, and they twinkle in anticipation of a person's reaction to what he is about to say. And it's hard to read Willis's age in his face. Despite the lines one would expect in someone "not ninety," his skin is remarkably fine-textured. Willis has a real face, undistorted by posturing or pretense. It is a face that belongs in a black-and-white photograph. To look upon it is to feel you have found some truth.

That day we moved quickly through the ritual of introduction and got to the issue at hand. "Willis," I told him, "don't mow my lawn this week."

"Oh, them there sheets won't bother me none. We'll fit right under them."

"But you do a lot of lawns, Willis. Just skip ours this week."

"Oh, no, can't do that. The grass gits too long, jams up in there under the mower, makes big clumps. Can't do that."

"Well, here's an idea. Why don't you mow everybody else's lawn first, and then, if there's still time, you can come back and do ours." I was, of course, counting on there not being enough time.

"Oh, no, that won't do. You see, I park my truck and then I unload my mower and we jest start in. Now, if I was to skip your lawn, I'd hafta load my mower up, drive it someplace else, do all that loadin' and unloadin' jest to git it back here. That won't do. Them there sheets won't bother me none."

"Oh, Willis, it isn't the sheets." I drew a deep breath. "I'll tell you the real reason I don't want you to mow the lawn." He studied me quietly while I tried to figure how best to present my case. "It's the violets, Willis." I gestured to the purple glory in the lawn behind him. He continued to stand facing me. "I have twelve guests coming for the weekend, and I want them to see those violets." Willis stood immobile. "Just look at them," I urged him. "Just turn around and look at how beautiful they are."

Dutifully Willis did my bidding, considering the display for an appropriate amount of time. Then he turned back, studying me as intently as he had the violets. He glanced briefly at his feet and then up at me. "Let me tell you somethin' about them there violets."

We stood facing each other silently. I understood that some response was expected. "What is that, Willis?"

"They're gonna die anyway."

Willis mowed my lawn that day. I told him that I didn't know why I hadn't thought of the imminent death of those violets myself. When he was finished, the lawn was a lovely, unremitting green.

In the years since our introduction, Willis has taught me much about violets and other things. But there are some things he leaves me to discover for myself. What he didn't tell me about the violets on our first meeting was that, although those in bloom were, indeed, on their way to death, there were others poised ready to blossom. Below the surface of his mower blade, short-stalked buds were waiting for just another day of sunshine to pull them to full magnificence of purple. By the time the weekend arrived, our guests were treated to a display of violets unlike any they had ever seen.

Birdsong reaches its glorious peak in May. I awake early enough to allow myself a charmed half hour. Lying quietly in bed, I rejoice in harmony. In our treetop, third-floor bedroom, we are surrounded by a loud, melodious choir of birds. It is a symphony made up of so many species and subspecies that I can't tease out the individual musicians. The first, barely audible chirps and whirrings don't really count as song. It's more like a tuning of instruments, a warming up. The first lyrical note is, I tell myself, a hermit thrush. But my ear is untrained and it could as easily be any other member of the thrush family, even one as common as the robin. That opening melody builds in intricate complexity as first one and then another joins the chorus. I visualize the cardinal conducting, for in the orchestrated pause his note rings clear and fluid, as if urging the others to join in to build to a full-throated, many-voiced pinnacle that gradually subsides to mere calls and twitters. They have ushered in the day and now return to the more mundane business of their lives.

I reluctantly abandon the brief respite from worry the feathered musicians have provided. I am fifty-four years old and sense that something is very wrong. Gene is snoring softly, evenly beside me. I run my right hand over my belly, not absentmindedly at all, but in pursuit of the twisted mass I know is waiting for me. "Diverticulitis" is what the young intern has told me. "It usually takes about three weeks for it to calm down. We'll schedule you for a colonoscopy at the end of the month. Call if you run a fever in the meantime."

I want to run a fever. This thing, whatever it is, is growing rapidly. Three weeks ago, it occupied only the lower left-hand quadrant of my abdomen. Now it fills my belly, reaching almost to my navel. Gene is awake. I reach over and take his hand, positioning it on the round knot just below my diaphragm. "What do you think it is," I ask, "a boy or a girl?"

"You scare me." He sounds helpless. Impatient too. Gene and I have different styles. I have been far less assertive with doctors than he would have been were he in a similar situation. "Shouldn't you give the hospital a call?"

"They said three weeks." Perhaps because I've often (and correctly) been called troublesome, I try to be careful about causing people trouble.

Gene is easing toward retirement. The first of this month, he moved to a three-day workweek. He now has four-day weekends. I keep to my regular schedule of writing and running, taking only Saturdays and Sundays off. It's Friday. Carol Feese, my friend and running partner, will be waiting for me at 7 A.M. on the road that circles around the lake. I stand up. I'm really not feeling very well, I'm plagued by some nameless malady, as if my intestines have locked up on me. I wonder if it is something I have eaten, and the thought of food of any kind sends a shudder through me. Perhaps this is the fever I've been waiting for.

I jam a thermometer between my teeth, close my lips tightly around it, and will the mercury to climb. I'm like a child hoping for a day off from school. The best I can do is ninety-nine degrees, high for me but nothing convincing enough for my mother to have allowed me to stay home. I always take Chuckles, our flat-coated retriever, with me when I run. I want to call the hospital, but I'm worried about how Chuckles and Gene will manage without me. Finally I call Carol and tell her the situation, my tentative decision not to run. She is jubilant. She's been urging me to get back in touch with the doctor whenever I report on the status of the ballooning mass in my belly.

Now I'm afraid the surgeon won't agree to let me come in. When the nurse asks my temperature, I fudge, "Just a little under a hundred." I don't expect her to be convinced, but perhaps she hears the panic in my voice. I've pulled it off. They'll be waiting for me. Gene takes Chuckles for a quick run while I shower and shave my legs. Do all women treat doctor's visits like assignations?

I'm surprised and relieved when they agree to admit me to the hospital, take it as proof that I'm not a hypochondriac, after all. Once in the hospital, I'm amazed at how easily I surrender responsibility. Gene will manage Chuckles and the cat. The doctors will manage the illness. They draw blood, order intravenous antibiotics, and promise a normal temperature by morning.

Serious faces greet me when I wake the next day. "There is no sign of infection in your blood."

I'm delighted. Picture myself going home. "Oh, great!"

"Not so great. It rules out diverticulitis. We've scheduled you for a CAT scan this afternoon."

Looking back on it, I guess I knew then. I think I really did know then, but I still was able to hold it all at bay, pretend that somehow there was some other reason. "Postmenopausal Woman Gives Birth to Twins." There is an inauthenticity to all the time that passed between that early-morning bedside conference and my moment of truth under the CAT scan. Most of that day was a lie. But the day has an importance, nonetheless. It marked the end of my false life.

I have since decided that it's hard for humans to know uncompromised joy until we face and accept our own death. And that day I was about to get my first lesson in mortality.

I'm playing a game with the CAT scan machine. I watch the digital readout and try to guess the intervals at which it will stop to take its pictures. Suddenly, the attendant reverses direction, backs up, and then rescans old territory. I feel myself tense. He repeats the procedure and then excuses himself for a few moments. When he returns, he tells me he is waiting for the surgeon to come down. I want to ask if this is standard procedure but don't want to put him on the spot. Dr. Rybeck arrives, makes the appropriate deliberations, and then comes and introduces himself. This is our first meeting. He stands beside me, his hand just barely touching my shoulder. "We're seeing quite a mass in your abdomen. I think it's ovarian in origin."

I interrupt him. "Are you telling me you think I have ovarian cancer?"

He nods. "Of course, we need to do more tests."

I start to cry. Gilda Radner springs to mind. "Don't tell me that one. That one's a killer. You know it is."

"I want to save you two surgeries. I've ordered a needle biopsy while we have you here under the CAT scan. A radiologist is coming right down. We should have the results back in a few days. Then we'll know exactly what we're dealing with. You're going to be staying in the hospital. We'll schedule surgery as soon as possible."

Whenever I've told this story to friends, they have reacted with horror at this doctor's abruptness. But I didn't see it that way then, and I don't see it that way now. His news was hard, but his honesty forged an immediate bond of trust. Here was a surgeon who sliced through the bullshit and went right to the heart of the matter. He cut all pretense away and planted my feet on a bedrock of honesty. I don't know if he was aware of it at the time, but those feet were already positioned in a fighter's stance. I hadn't yet formed my hands into fists, but the day was coming when I would.

There are no surprises in the lab report. It is ovarian cancer. My medical education is beginning. It is undifferentiated, primitive, rapidly growing. Carol, Gene, and I could have told them the rapidly growing part. Because it is ovarian cancer, I am being reassigned, out of general surgery and into gynecological oncology. My new surgeon, Dr. Strider, gives me the good news and the bad news on undifferentiated cancer. Mine has already spread so far that he knows even before opening me up that he is not going to be able to remove it all. "We'll do what we call a debulking. The goal is to leave you with no tumors larger than a nickel. The chemotherapy has a good chance of being effective on tumors that size and smaller. Rapidly growing tumors respond better to chemo than slowly growing ones. But it's all a wash when it comes to your chances for survival." I understand that in the recovery period between surgery and the first chemotherapy treatment, my rapidly growing tumors may become too large to respond.

I like Dr. Strider, my new surgeon, very much. He and Dr. Rybeck have honesty in common; beyond that, however, their styles are very different. Dr. Strider always makes me laugh. He never comes into the room without a smile. He feels like a friend who is interested in me as a person. He makes the mistake of asking me about the book I am writing, *Sex and the Single Tax*, and I launch an immediate campaign to make him see the wisdom of taxing all natural resources, especially land. The American economist Henry George developed this theory over a hundred years ago. I want Dr. Strider to understand how its implementation could eliminate the growing disparity between rich and poor. It is the start of many bedside discussions. I'm eager to show him that I have important work to do in this world. I want to be someone worth saving. I can't help feeling my life hangs on my skill in debate.

I am unaware of it at the time, but I am already bargaining with the gods. I make quick judgments about what I am willing to surrender and what I wish to keep. They can have almost all body parts. My brain, however, is off-limits. The uterus, ovaries, appendix, can and will go. I wasn't using them anyway. Omentum, major and minor? Take them. How can I be attached to something I didn't even know I had until yesterday? Peritoneum, diaphragm, intestines? Go ahead, pluck tumors at will, although, having an unfortunate discomfort with body functions, I fervently hope I wake from surgery spared the potential colostomy. But I really know that I have taken a gambler's desperate last stance when they tell me they have scheduled surgery for May 27, and my first reaction is one of relief. Only later do I remember the violets. I have given up on all those flowers without protest. My spirit is broken. The violets will have to bloom without me this year.

The death that has touched me most deeply is a death I never knew or at least never experienced directly. My mother's mother died when Mother was seven, leaving her essentially responsible for two younger brothers. Only after Mother's own death at eighty did I learn all the cruel details surrounding that first death. Her father almost immediately left his three small children with relatives and ran off to marry another woman. Mother never spoke to me of this shadowy other wife, a silence that was made easy by the fact that Granddaddy abandoned her and their three sons as well. The Carberry clan formed a wall of secrecy around the whole scandal, a wall so effective that his second wife was never able to locate him, and I grew up not realizing I had hidden uncles.

I don't know which has affected me most, the parts of the story I was told or the parts that were left out. Mother had no time for self-pity. Her tales of her mother's death were beautifully rendered, mythic fairy tales, sweet and sad. Jennie, radiant Jennie, lay dying in a white, gauzelike tent erected in the backyard to give her the benefit of fresh air. Each afternoon, Mother and her two little brothers were brought to the bedside to visit with their frail and fading mama. My mother was always vague about the cause of death, something consumptive and wasting, taking life but leaving beauty there.

And Jennie was beautiful. Since childhood, I've studied the surviving photos. Such as Jennie at the beach with her firstborn, my mother, then a laughing toddler, both of them filled with joy. I was as drawn to the photos as I was haunted by the sense of an unwanted psychic vision. For I already knew the ending to this tender maternal scene: there were to be no happily ever afters.

All the deaths that followed this one in my life have had an unreal quality, since they fail to match the romantic standard of billowing white fabric, a curtain drawn between this heroic, flawless creature and her three babies.

Chapter 2

June

It is hard for someone who has been raised on melodramatic fairy tales to surrender instantly the maudlin potential of a major illness. I am a fighter, of course I am, but there are moments, I have to admit, in which death has its appeal. It's as if I get to write my own romantic ending. It's a way of sanitizing my life, erasing all the flaws, the fights, the troublesome aspects of my character. I want a moon-filled diaphanous tent. I want to fade beautifully into freshly laundered white bed linens. I want my children gathered round while I drift off into perfection uncontaminated by the messy business of life. I think of my grandfather's vanishing act and can't script a well-defined part for Gene in this little one-act play. Will I be so easily forgotten? Is there someone waiting in the wings, poised to take my place, to fill my role? Can one person be so easily substituted for another?

It's the first day of June. I've got a belly held together by a row of staples that runs from my diaphragm to my pubic bone. This is not exactly the stuff of romance. Do I want to live or do I want to die? It's becoming pretty clear that white tents are not standard hospital supply. The various stomach and IV tubes are a pretty poor substitute. I can't stand looking like a sick person. I hate all this medical equipment sticking out of my nose and arms. I plead desperately with the nurses to pull all the tubes out before the start of visiting hours. No one I love is going to see me looking like this. "I can swallow that NG tube again. I can. I can. I don't mind doing it." They give me no sympathy, insist my family members can handle it, and, of course, they are right.

Still, it is hard for me to see all the fear and sadness in my loved ones' eyes. Other than Gene, Ingrid is my first visitor. She comes up from Philadelphia right away. She moves quietly into the room. "Hi, Mommy." Responding to my passion for fresh fruit, she's made a lovely ceramic bowl and filled it to the brim with the season's first sweet, dark oxheart cherries. Gene has been vague about medical details. No one has told Ingrid that I am unable to eat. She hesitates and looks just slightly stricken while I explain that it will be awhile before I can take anything by mouth. "But the bowl is beautiful," I tell her.

She recovers quickly. " 'The Gift of the Magi,' " she says, referring to O. Henry's short story. We both laugh.

"They smell good. Who says you have to eat cherries?" I ask. "Some people just like to smell them." The two of us bend our heads over the bowl and inhale the fresh, fruity aroma. We exclaim over their polished, near-black gleam. I ask her about the bowl, and she shows me how she has glazed the rim only, leaving the red clay interior unpainted so that it will draw off any moisture left from washing. "Don't worry," she tells me. "I'll bring you more cherries when you come home. For now, these will lure the nurses into your room. You know they must get tired of bedside chocolates."

Gene and I are blessed with a family both emotionally and geographically close. In another June, two years ago, two years before this illness taught me that June can carry other than joy, my son, Craig, his wife, Dee, and their three-year-old daughter, Erin, followed us to Osprey Lakes. They've since had another child. Kyle, now ten months old, rounds out the little family. How brave they were to pull up stakes and move to Sullivan County where the local economy makes earning a living a dicey proposition at best. Before the move, Craig had been a cowboy, a herdsman, tending purebred Angus cattle. Purebred-cattle raising is the hobby of the very wealthy. Although financial comfort is descriptive of this rural county's summer population, its year-round farmers work the earth and not the IRS. Always skilled with his hands, Craig found a new vocation with a local contractor and learned a carpenter's trade while employed to help in the construction of his own log home. Dee did interim work as a waitress while she readied herself for an eventual career in real estate. But most of all, they brought us Erin and Kyle. And now, their presence here is a godsend for both Gene and me. Even when Gene is working in Philadelphia, I will have kin within a half mile of my home, ready for emergency call.

Still, the hardest visit of all is when Craig and Dee bring those two darling babies in to see me. Kyle, of course, is too little to be anything but fascinated by the workings of IV tubes. He grins and laughs as his chubby fingers with their dimpled knuckles reach to grab the dangling equipment. He is too young to understand that his grandmother is sick. Dear Erin is a different story. Erin has always had her own style, and it starts with sizzle. Today, however, she holds back and requires atypical prompting before handing me the get-well card she has made. Her large green eyes are solemn. I am totally unprepared for how unclean I feel. "I can't kiss them," I whisper to Craig. "I don't want to contaminate them." I know it is irrational. I know cancer isn't contagious, but I see even my hands as skeletal, reaching, pulling them toward some dank sepulchral place. Theirs is an innocence I want left untouched. But having failed as a protector, my own dark shadow casts the promise of mortality across their previously unblemished cheeks.

By the time Gene's daughter, Dana, and her husband, Derek, show up with our two other grandchildren, I've had time to forewarn myself and them. It is no lack of love that keeps me from touching Cody, only six or seven weeks old, and Leighanne, not yet two. It is a chill fear that I will somehow draw them into this out-of-season funeral march.

When one of the doctors first told me I had cancer, I protested, "I'm too young!" If he at thirty-something found my fifty-something protests amusing, he did not let on. "Lots of women much younger than you are diagnosed with cancer."

No one in my family, myself included, had ever seen me as a potential candidate for cancer. There is no family history. I eat lots of fruits, vegetables, and whole grains. I exercise. I laugh. I've never smoked and drink so little that my reaction to even one glass of wine is something of a joke among my friends. When I first felt the lumps that later proved to be my undoing, I voiced the obvious fear to Craig. "Oh, Mom," he reassured me. "Don't worry. You're not the type to get cancer." So, a week ago when I called from the hospital to tell him the unpleasant truth, there was a long silence on the other end of the line. I heard him sigh. And then, finally, he made his pronouncement: "Oh, boy, that poor cancer is going to find out it picked on the wrong body this time."

I have a reputation to live up to, and much as I might want to take the easy way out, it is becoming increasingly difficult to consider death as a serious option. I am discovering that I do, indeed, want to live. Still, I am realistic. I know I am up against tremendous odds. I find myself bouncing around all over the place. "I'm going to beat this" is what I tell all those who love me, but I don't always believe it. I spend my mornings trying calmly to ready myself for death, but by afternoon I am busy plotting strategies to fight off this stealthy coward. I know I hate being sick. If it can't be a white-tent kind of death, I'm not signing on. My friends and family are great. Within hours of my diagnosis, they started rallying around me, and they haven't let up since. I have O negative blood. When Dave, the owner of my favorite hardware store, hears I need additional transfusions, he is there to offer up a wholesome, homegrown product. I complain about the horror of hospital gowns, and Carol, using sexy Victoria's Secret pajamas as a pattern, stitches together a pair with Velcro side and shoulder seams. Dee's friend Susan Mathias sends in fluffy, spike-heeled, white mules, absolutely contraindicated for walking, but great for dangling off the toe of my foot as I lie in bed.

I don't want to die, the timing is wrong. But what if I'm going to die anyhow? What then? True to my sister's childhood assessment, in those moments when my near-immediate demise seems the most likely outcome, I soften the blow by telling myself the whole scenario is the answer to some old, former-life prayer. Sandy would find it predictable that I insist this is all something I really wanted to happen. I decide I probably need a cancer death and just hope it won't be too painful and that I will learn something from the experience. I don't subscribe to any formal religious doctrine and can't explain why, against all intellectual arguments with myself, I almost always have had a stubborn belief in reincarnation. Years ago I decided that it didn't matter if souls were actually recycled or whether this was just some comfort my brain manufactured in response to the ego's inability to comprehend nonexistence. The creed seemed a practical way to govern one's life.

Never having studied Eastern religions, I have only a pop-culture understanding of karma, enlightenment, nirvana. However, a belief that I will have to keep repeating a mistake until I finally get it right is powerful incentive to aspire to fairness and honesty in my daily dealings. When faced with a difficult moral choice, I often buck up my conscience by telling my-self, "Learn your lesson now. The next time around, the classroom might not be nearly as comfortable." I can't pretend that I always heed my own advice. When temptation is strong enough, I am able to rationalize that I am simply guaranteeing further lifetimes. And isn't life, complete with all its gritty aspects, more fun than some free-form and ultimately boring nirvana? Floating in this bastardized amalgam of beliefs is a notion that in the moments immediately following my death, I, unburdened by either guilt or defensiveness, will get to review my own life. While in that state, I will be able to see what it is I still need to learn and will therefore select my next life with an eye to the situations that best give me an opportunity to learn it.

Denial is generally considered the first stage of reaction when faced with death. I suppose there is something of denial in my repeated insistence that this near guarantee of death from cancer is my own very clever choice. Well, if it is denial, it is my morning form of the condition. The afternoon variety is characterized by negotiation. "Look," I say to whatever powers there be, "I don't see why it's necessary for me to actually have to *die* of cancer. I can probably learn really a lot just by being awfully sick, just by *thinking* I'm going to die of cancer."

I am surrounded with books and five-by-eight cards. Notes for my project on precolonial systems of land tenure compete with me for bed space. I am determined to use these two weeks in the hospital as working hours. But I keep drifting off into dream-filled sleep. I awake from one such dream filled with a sense of mission and purpose. I am certain that everything I have written so far is wrong and must be discarded. My approach has been far too flippant. *Sex and the Single Tax,* indeed! From now on the book shall be called *Out of England,* the title a bitter play on Isak Dinesen's romantic account of British colonial presence. My own view is darker. I can't make a joke of the economic distortion that began with the English Enclosure Acts and continues to fuel the growing disparity between rich and poor. I become convinced that, contrary to my first idea, it is dishonest to pull a literary bait and switch, luring readers with a promise of sex only to offer them land-value taxation. I burn with the desire to get to the typewriter and begin again. Finishing my book becomes my reason for being, a point I will not negotiate. I have to live until I finish the book. And how clever of me to insist on starting over with chapter one. Writing for time.

Now that I have the terms established, I am eager to get home. I've run through five roommates, all but one of them cancer patients. I'm beginning to feel unfairly confined, locked up for a crime I didn't commit. I stand staring out metal-framed windows, unable to see much but other wings of the hospital. Only in the distance can I glimpse traces of a far-off mountain. Hanging to my IV pole, I pace the hospital corridors. When I can't sleep in the middle of the night, I get up and walk. So determined am I to get some mileage in that one young intern, himself a runner, recognizes the signs of an exercise addict and threatens to keep me in the hospital until my incision is completely healed. "I'm telling you, if you run before that's completely healed, it won't be a pretty sight. Guts all over the sidewalk."

I am starved for fresh air. Unable to sleep without the windows flung wide open, I feel trapped by technology. Even my dreams carry the theme. In my most vivid one, I am a fish pinned to a wooden dock by a stainless steel spike. All around me, my beloved lake beckons, its waters dancing and sparkling in the sun. Green leaves wave silhouetted by the blue of summer sky. I struggle against the nail that holds me fast and, in my thrashing, drive sharp splinters through my scales. My eyeballs become dry and shrunken like those of fish that have lain too long on ice in a supermarket cooler. I understand that I am done. Waking from this dream, I want to crash the IV pole against the wall and break loose from all that holds me here.

When they finally agree to release me, the decision is a sudden one. Gene is in Philadelphia. Carol comes to drive me home. The hospital doors close behind us, and I feel that I am seeing the world for the first time. The colors are so intense that tears fill my eyes. My throat catches. A whole season has passed without me. When I came into the hospital, leaves were just forming, and now it is full-blown summer.

The fifty-minute drive from the hospital to Osprey Lakes is over roads that curve and wind through green fields and rolling hills. Oriental poppies bloom scarlet-orange in overgrown gardens. I think I have never seen so many shades of green. The beech leaves are nearly liquid, so intense that they seem to contain their own source of light. I have forgotten how green new green can be. There is already a lazy summer feel. Daisies and orchid-colored spheres of dame's rocket crowd the roadsides. The sky is bright blue and filled with white, high-floating clouds. Carol and I are giddy with laughter. Our morning runs have been filled with a shared appreciation of the natural world, and now I feel that I have already exhausted all the superlatives and have nothing left to express my joy in the glimmering perfection of this day.

Only when we ease into the village of Osprey Lakes itself does reality slice through my happiness. The Sweet Shop is open and a small group of laughing vacationers, ice cream cones in hand, wander across in front of our car. The frame freezes, and I am struck through with envy. Their care-free, smiling chatter is from another world, part of a life I've left behind. It is from a place so far from where I now live that it feels gone from me forever. I sense that I have become a tourist in my own land and feel that the native language is lost to me, that I no longer speak the dialect. Joy is easy, easier perhaps than ever, but the unquestioning belief that one day will follow another has completely vanished.

Time will pass. Months will pass, but that moment will stay with me. It truly is the first and only occasion I've had anything close to a "Why me?" reaction. I won't have the feeling again, but neither will I forget that relaxed group and the dislocation engendered by their laughter.

When I was first diagnosed, my children and some of my friends did ask, "Why you?" My answer was always an honest "Why not me?" This disease seemed a fitting judgment on someone who took such a vocal populist stance. What could possibly be more democratic than cancer? The incidence may be democratic. The treatment hardly is. When I was presented with the first $1,700 bill for a ten-day supply of a prescription drug, I was forced to acknowledge the privileges conferred by our economic status. Survival of the fittest? Perhaps, as long as calculations of fitness include a firm reckoning of the bottom line.

Carol is reluctant to leave me alone. I sense in her an unspoken condemnation of Gene, and I struggle to make her understand. It is hard to explain, even to someone who knows us both. One of the things I most love about Gene is his understanding of my need for solitude. "I love people, but I require solitude" is my standard line. But unless one has lived with me, it is impossible to communicate how deep that lonely river runs. Especially now. Now more than ever I crave an existence uncluttered by people. The truth is hard, a side of myself I would rather not expose. I simply *need* to be alone. I feel truly safe only when alone.

Of course, I'm not really alone. Chuckles is waiting at the door. Once Gene's two-week vacation time was over, Craig and Dee took over dog duty. They brought Chuckles home this afternoon, and he is contorted in a funny mix that looks to contain elements of both joy and chagrin. He greets me with uncharacteristic gentleness. I had feared great bounding leaps that would eviscerate me on the way down. Instead, he wags his whole body but keeps an almost slinking posture as he smells me all over. Flat-coated retrievers are big, long-haired dogs. Chuckles weighs eighty-five pounds. Unfortunately, his physical strength has not been matched by restraint. He looks like a dog but acts like a puppy. Except for his black coat, he could be mistaken for a golden retriever on speed; however, today he impresses me with what appears to be a genuine sensitivity to my frail state.

The house is lovely, cool, and welcoming. Dee has cleaned. No speck of dust or dog-nose print on the window distracts me from the serene comfort offered here. My own place. My own space. My own quiet. No ever-present TV game shows, no loudspeakered hospital codes. No medicinal nor antiseptic smells. Just home. Dee has made a bed for me on the couch in front of the fireplace. Stairs are off-limits for a while. The sheets are white and crisp, sweet repositories of summer sun and mountain air. I don't care that it's the middle of the day. I want nothing more than sleep.

When I wake, I discover that I have a new "nurse," and he has been busy. Chuckles has taken every toy from his toy box and jammed them in around my sleeping form. There is a stuffed rabbit under my chin. A small basketball is wedged between my left ear and the couch. A half-chewed rawhide bone is at the top of my head. My feet are surrounded by small items: a little yellow duck with a squeaker, several tennis balls, and a woebegone stuffed squirrel that he inherited from his predecessor. The crowning touch is a Frisbee on my stomach. I can't decide if these are gifts or reminders that I owe him some play time!

This sweet, comical dog has joined the forces that work to urge me back to health. The toys-while-sleeping routine is one that he will continue until I am strong enough to move to one of the bedrooms on the second floor. He deposits them so gently that he never wakes me, and I can only guess at what is going on in his mind. Is this some flat-coated burial rite? Has he been watching TV specials on Egyptian pharaohs? I choose to interpret the behavior as an act of love, an expression of the deep but unspoken bond between dogs and their humans.

Before I left the hospital, the running doctor reminded me that daily jogs were off-limits for a while. "But I can walk, right?" I asked him. "You're already walking," he responded.

Now as I get ready to take Chuckles for his afternoon constitutional on my first day home, I wonder if that doctor understood what I meant by walking. I briefly consider abandoning my ritual hike on the Laurel Path, which circles our lake. The terrain is rough and my footing not that steady. However, the alternative is even more treacherous. Walking through town with an eighty-five-pound wild thing lunging joyously at the end of the lead cannot possibly be what the doctor had in mind. Off-lead on the Laurel Path seems the safest solution. We won't go all the way around. I intend to gradually increase the length of these out-and-back ventures until I am once more back to the old routine.

The Laurel Path is always near-hypnotic in its power to soothe and restore me. Old photographs from our town's Victorian heyday show the trail to be essentially unchanged. Some wisdom and deep appreciation for the unaltered beauty of the natural state inspired the early founders to set aside a preserve completely encircling the lake. No property may come within one hundred feet of the shoreline. As a result, only the handful of docks and boathouses that were erected prior to the formation of the Lake Association detract from an unspoiled view of mountain laurel, hemlock, and native rhododendron reaching out over crystal-clear water in an unbroken sweep. Today blueberry bushes, heavy with bloom and a sweet fragrance that hints at the coming harvest, are clustered around the arching footbridge that spans the divide between outlet pond and lake. I am home.

It has been years since I have gone to church, but the lake and the woods circling it have a holy splendor. There is one spot that I have always quite privately called my temple. Today, Chuckles and I will walk that far before we turn around. There are places where the trees fall back, and for just a moment, the path becomes the shore. This hour before dusk is caught with stillness. The surface of the water is so calm that my eye is drawn to the slightest hint of movement. The dorsal fin of a passing fish briefly ripples the mirrored glass, then all is motionless once more, clouds and trees in matched perfection in the lake and against the sky.

Although the path twists over roots and outcroppings of rock, my foot falls quietly on a cushion of pine needles and wood chips. As we enter the tall stand of ancient hemlock that marks the cathedraled entrance to my holy place, the flutelike call of a thrush heralds approaching evening. The lower trucks of these trees catch the sun only at the first and last light of day. As a result, they reach tall and free of branches for at least thirty feet. Long, unbroken shadows reflect no movement and give the illusion of time briefly frozen. Eons ago glaciers sculpted a semicircular cliff that captures this wooded hollow and holds it apart from the world at large.

The path winds just slightly uphill, curving through some rhododendron and away from the silent trees. In years past, one of their sisters fell and blocked the trail. A cross-section of the trunk, three feet in diameter and just wide enough to allow passage single file, was sawed out and removed. Progressive seasons of weather have given this fallen giant soft edges. Gentle decay in russet tones of chestnut returns it to the earth.

To one side, a cluster of small maple trees, no more than eighteen inches high, gives testimony to the transforming but enduring nature of the forest. When I first came to Osprey Lakes, I claimed one of these little trees as my bush soul. Or, rather, it claimed me. Months from now, Ingrid will challenge my choice of an arboreal soul mate.

"Couldn't you have chosen something a little sturdier, in a more protected spot?"

Certainly it is true that this little tree is perilously close to the path and easily stepped upon. In the fall, the clear scarlet of its leaves has on at least two occasions inspired someone to break off small branches. I don't know why this particular tree called out to me. Perhaps it was its very vulnerability. But I don't tell Ingrid that. I hear her unspoken fear.

"Don't worry. I won't give up and die if the tree does." My answer is easy, but it speaks to Ingrid's heart and doesn't really come from my own. The truth I feel is that it doesn't matter. This tree and I are bound in a way that has nothing to do with objective assessments of life and death.

Just beyond the little maple tree is a wall of layered rock, cleft by a small spring. This spot is the temple's center. It is cool here on the hottest day of summer. The spring is a bit of a foul-weather friend, flowing freely only at the end of winter or following a heavy rain. But even though its waterfall is not reliably raging and spectacular, there is always some moisture to be harvested here. The stratified sandstone face is struck through with muted shades of copper, green, and gray. Dense moss holds tiny beads of water. I touch my fingertips to these and rub cool dew across my cheeks and forehead. Feeling blessed by this humble ritual, I turn and head back to the house with Chuckles.

Someone tells me that when Willis was informed I had cancer, he sat in his truck and cried. I've been home from the hospital only a few days when he comes to visit. Gene lets him in. Willis sits and chats awkwardly. I keep telling him I'm going to be fine, but lying drowsy on the couch, I'm aware I don't paint a convincing picture. I inquire about Willis's wife, Mabel. I've learned her name from others. Willis refers to her, with near-biblical reverence, only as "the woman." We both try to steer the conversation away from illness, but it is not so easily led. No matter what question we raise, the answer reminds us both of some health-related issue. Never having been sick and, until now, unschooled in surgical technique, I am fascinated by the row of metal staples that sutures my belly together. It looks as if some carpenter went wild with a staple gun and outfitted me with a tiny railroad track that runs from stem to stern. Tiny railroad tracks or a giant zipper, whatever it is, it looks to have more to do with a mechanic's trade than with a surgeon's. As Willis gets up to leave, I impulsively ask him if he'd like to see this work of art. After all, if Lyndon Johnson could show an entire press corps his scar, I guess I can show Willis mine.

Willis protests, but he peers over the back of the couch as I lift my shirt to reveal the gleaming metal. He seems suitably impressed, but it is only as he heads out the door that I learn the reason.

"You're tough," he says in awe. "The woman won't show ya nothin'."

I am scheduled for my first chemotherapy treatment toward the end of the month. Try as I might to focus on other things, predictably I am preoccupied with thoughts of cancer. It is the first thing that runs through my mind when I wake in the morning and is firmly lodged in my brain even as I fall uneasily to sleep. I picture the growing tumors on my intestines and diaphragm and try to will them gone. I harbor this brooding undercurrent even when Gene and I sit and chat, ostensibly of other things. In many ways it is easier when he is in Philadelphia. Then I can just give myself over to this romance with death.

Romance is too strong a word. Things have not progressed that far. It is a little flirtation I have going here. There is a lot of circling, approach/avoidance kind of silliness. This dark fellow is a wonderfully seductive suitor, but I am feeling coy, unwilling to commit to terms so final. Still the appeal is there. Expertise is a powerful aphrodisiac, and he does tempt me with sweet promises: "You don't know what you're missing. Try it and your life never again will be the same." No arguing with that one, but it is too reminiscent of lines I have heard before. "Until you have known me, you can't know life," he whispers in my ear. Charnel knowledge, bliss of bliss, all questions answered, but there is something of the lothario here. He's coming on too fast, and I draw back, lower my lashes, stall for time. "Thanks all the same," I tell him. "I think we need to get to know each other a little better."

Gene and I sit in the oncology waiting room. It's our first time here. Surgery is dramatic. It feels like the major battle in a front-page war. Chemotherapy is mud-and-blood-in-the-trenches maneuvering in a country nobody really wants to hear about. I'm anxious about how I'll hold up over the long haul of the months ahead and surreptitiously stare at the other people gathered here. I play a game. Which one is the patient, which one the worried relative? Bald heads let me fill in the first blanks quickly. Still, there are some tough cases here. Needing more clues, I strain to eavesdrop on conversations, most of them surprisingly mundane. It's easy when you catch them coming in.

The name on the file folder is a dead giveaway, so to speak. I marvel at the thickness of most files; New York telephone-book size is not uncommon. Wide rubber bands hold clusters of smaller manila folders together, all of them belonging to a single person. My own is still comparatively thin. The nurses greet most folks by name on sight. They tease with one man about his loud jacket. So much laughter. I don't feel inclined to join in. Gene and I are unusually silent, not much to say really, so we just sit and wait my turn.

Dr. Silverman will be my guide through this chemical rite of passage. I've met him just briefly once before. He came to my bedside and introduced himself. I was a bit disappointed. The anthropologist in me wanted a little flash and glitter, some shaking of rattles, feathers, thumb-drawn lines of black and ocher paint across the cheekbones, perhaps a fancy dance step or two. This medicine man is clearly a man of science, and I'm not sure science is going to be enough. He talks in medical statistics. He explains the drugs and lists the possible side effects in terms of probability. He is thorough. We ask a few questions. He gives answers. There seems to be surprisingly little that either Gene or I want to say. Finally, he checks my vital signs, and I am cleared for takeoff, all systems go.

The chemotherapy room itself is hideous. Layered with dull green paint, it is a windowless vault hidden in the hospital basement, life's dirty little secret. The walls are lined with about a dozen reclining chairs, each one equipped with the requisite IV pole. Some kind of Naugahyde upholstery covers these beds disguised as chairs, ease of cleanup an obvious factor here. Curtains can be pulled for privacy. A TV drones on, talk show, game show, soap opera, least-common-denominator television. I don't think I belong here, don't really feel like staying. Ingrid, cleverly suspecting the worst, has given me a headset and pocket-size tape player and a tape, *Puccini without Words*. I'm surprised at how very sick everyone looks. Some people smell very sick. There's not much hair in sight, a few bad wigs. One woman in a hospital gown has been rolled in on a bed to receive her treatment. Another is so emaciated that I can't help but stare. In here, it's real easy to tell the patients from the relatives.

My "lounge chair" is in the corner. Between me and the man next to us, Gene sits down in the straight-backed version provided for friends and relations. My conversational skills have deserted me. All I can do is glance around the room and think, "Is this what I'm going to look like in six months?" My poor veins are already so scarred that the IV nurses must move up through the ranks before someone is finally able to hit a vein that doesn't roll. I suspect myself of deliberately holding out, although I do what I'm told and extend my arm in apparent compliance with all requests. It is decided I will have a Mediport inserted before my next scheduled visit to the chemo room. Gene asks if I'm okay. I don't answer, just nod yes. He tries to chat with me, but I can't find much to say. The folks beside us have no such problem. Gene is a clown. Soon he is telling jokes and funny stories. He keeps them laughing. The wife, the healthy member of the team, asks about the duration of my treatments.

I answer, "Not long, I hope. Six months if all goes well."

Her husband laughs. "Don't count on that, but it's not so bad. I'll be in here every week, once a week, for the rest of my life. Everybody knows me here."

I slip the headset on, crank up Puccini, feign sleep, and turn my face to the wall so no one can see the tears squeezing out between closed lids.

When I was five, my sisters and I enjoyed an amount of independence unheard of for youngsters in the nineties. We moved in a pack of other kids. An informal maternal network kept behind-the-scenes watch, and there was a great sense of security as long as we stayed on our own side of the block. The other side of the block was a different story. Those few older kids who had been brave enough to venture over there came back with tales of boys with sticks, a nation of bullies.

The safety net of peers and mothers failed me one day, I don't remember how. I just have this image of myself sitting tied up in a little red express wagon while the three bullies pulled me to their home base on the forbidden side of the block. I don't know why I didn't scream. As they threatened me with promises of torture, I silently planned my escape. When they began arguing among themselves over where to take me, I seized on the division in their ranks to offer a compromise plan: "If you'll take me home, I'll give you all my money."

They quickly forgot their disagreement over the appropriate site for torture and coalesced around this novel idea of kidnap for ransom. Back to my house we went. They stopped the wagon by my front steps and said, "Go get your money."

"You'll have to untie me first." I don't think they had thought of this. Bullies are not always known for their brains. As soon as my feet touched the sidewalk, I sprinted for my front door. With my hand safely on the latch, I called over my shoulder, "Ha, ha, ha! I don't have any money!"

That was true. I didn't have any money. But help me with this moral issue: Is a promise to surrender all my money a statement that I actually have some?

Chapter 3

July

I'm struggling with a dilemma. I've asked for enough time to finish my book. I've already extended the time required from six months to twelve. Is it too late to introduce another dimension here? It's pretty important to me that I live long enough that my grandchildren will remember me. Cody is newly born. I figure I'm talking five years or so, depending on his language skills. And Ingrid, my oldest child, has postponed marriage and childbearing into some unspecified future. I certainly intend to know her children and want them to have some sense of me. I'm beginning to regret committing to shorter terms than I'm now willing to honor. Is asking for a year the same as promising to die when that year is up? I decide that it is not, but am troubled by an uncomfortable sense that I'm up to my old tricks.

July in Osprey Lakes makes me understand why most people love summer. (I'm more of a winter person, myself. It plays to my darker side.) But July here is rich with the textures and sounds of lazy summer happiness. Arched tunnels of native rhododendron bloom pale and ephemeral along the Laurel Path. The relaxed laughter of children at play drifts across the lawns. The distant hum of Willis's mower forms a backdrop for ice tinkling in glasses.

Soft conversation. The slamming of the Sweet Shop door. Blessedly sound-less sailboats tacking with billowing sails across the lake. (No motorboats for Osprey Lakes.) The canoes are mostly ancient wooden Old Towns. Not even the slap of waves against an aluminum hull disturbs the sense of old-fashioned summer days.

There is the sweet sense of being caught in a time warp, lost, perhaps, in the late forties. No one worries about crime. War and political strife seem to be located on another planet. Here, there is just the beach, the old bath-houses with their blackened cedar shakes and dark green trim, and the last of the mountain laurel blooming in sticky pink and white glory. Seventy-two degrees seems to be about as warm as the lake ever gets, and it might be the end of the month before that happens. The water is clear all the way to the bottom. I like to swim out to the floating dock, heave myself out of the lake with all the grace of an aging sea elephant, and just lie there, so charmed by the gentle rocking motion and the warmth of the sun that I hesitate to breathe for fear of breaking the spell.

The Fourth of July parade is a little slice of Norman Rockwell's Amer-ica. It begins at the old fire hall and community center and ends at the vil-lage green, about three and a half blocks away. Short blocks. Blink and you'll miss it, but almost nobody does. The children, summer and year-round res-idents alike, gather at the starting place an hour before the appointed time to decorate tricycles, bikes, little red wagons, dogs, and themselves. Free crepe paper, Scotch tape, and advice are equally available to everyone. There is no contest, just celebration, democracy at its best, a level playing field (at least for those already privileged enough to be here). Most of the dogs are wear-ing clothing. Red, white, and blue is the major color theme for dogs and people alike. Gene worried the year I had Chuckles carry a flag, was afraid some patriots might be offended if he dragged it. But true to his retriever her-itage, he marched with head held high, the little flag safe above the ground. Sometimes a big dog or small pony will pull a cart loaded with a giggling crop of blondies so obviously dipped from the same gene pool that every-one knows they are some grandfather's pride and joy.

Half the town marches in the parade and the other half watches. As far as I'm concerned, those who are off playing golf during this spectacle can't re-ally be counted as bona fide citizens of Osprey Lakes. We don't have a band—we don't need one. A recording of John Philip Sousa blares from the opened window of the van carrying Penelope Curtis. Penny, wrapped in an American flag, clings to the luggage rack. Every now and then, her husband leans out the car window and asks the crowd at large, "Is she still up there?" Although Penelope is in her eighties, she has the best legs in town, and the flag is strategically draped to show them to full advantage.

We may not have a band, but we do have a drum major. Ray Schrecken-gast and the Osprey Lakes Athletic Association run a wonderful and varied summer program for the children. Should the kids choose to participate, there is something to keep them busy all day long. Today, however, Ray's job is to lead the parade. Wearing a towering drum major's hat/helmet, he marches ahead banging the beat on a bass drum. Members of the volunteer fire company hang off our antique fire engine and throw candy into the crowd. Gene, not to be outdone by Penelope Curtis, kicks his way along on a child's scooter while dressed as Superman. Superman? On the Fourth of July? Somehow it all works in the Osprey Lakes parade.

Craig and Dee had two dogs, Vern and Casey, when they first moved here. Vern was a huge, slow-moving Newfoundland who kept Casey, affec-tionately referred to as Space Casey, in line. That year, when Vern and his springer spaniel sidekick marched in the parade, all comment was reserved for lumbering Vern. Unfortunately, Vern, like other large breeds, had a life span of only nine years. With Vern's death, Casey was released from his role of straight man and came fully into his own. Craig and Dee, busy with jobs and small children, were dismayed to find that the "new" Casey had an in-dependent streak when it came to leash laws. He could slip through a screen door in a flash, dive into the cover of the ferns at the first turn of a head, and be off and on his way to the beach.

Sometimes when Gene and I would be walking Chuckles on the Laurel Path, we'd bump into Casey, off on an adventure. "Watch out! He's got his sunglasses and beach towel," Gene would say, laughing. And it was true. There was no denying his intent. Which would all be well and good, except that dogs, somehow deemed less sanitary than people, are forbidden in the lake, and there are those who take our leash laws mighty seriously. When Casey saw us, you could almost hear him mutter, "Oops." He knew the drill; we would turn him around and take him back home. As a result, Casey be-came ever more sophisticated in his technique. He would lie in wait along the path until some unsuspecting family walked by, and then he would attach himself to the little group with a bond that could only have been born of a lifetime of devotion. Now when he saw us, he would cut us dead, claiming never to have met us before in his life. People were bewildered. "He's not our dog," they would tell us, but they were always slightly embarrassed. How could they possibly be telling the truth? Casey's perfect "heel" could have come only from years of practice.

The first time Craig walked Casey in the parade sans Vern, he deeply regretted having failed to hang a sign around Casey's neck that read, "Lost dog. Found at the beach," because as the two of them marched by, group after group could be heard saying, "Oh, so that's whose dog that is."

After the parade, the whole town gathers for a sweetly patriotic speech and prayer by one of the ministers who serve the needs of our summer community. There are three lovely old churches that are fully operational only during July and August. Cookies and lemonade are served to the children on the back lawn of the Voorhees place, a big Victorian home that borders the village green and the lake. My favorite description of the Fourth of July in Osprey Lakes was penned by a travel writer for the *Philadelphia Inquirer*. He claimed that ours was the kind of parade that Tom Sawyer would have designed if he'd been from old money.

I'm feeling surprisingly good. The first chemotherapy treatment left me well enough to attend a cocktail party a few days afterward. I still can't run, but I'm walking the whole way around the lake, two miles, morning and night. And I'm delighting in the outpouring of affection from family and friends. My promise to beat this thing begins to have a more genuine ring to it. Ingrid comes up almost every weekend. She tempts my less than robust appetite with all kinds of health-filled magic from the blender. She washes sheets and makes beds and brings funny videos, available only in the city. Norman Cousins has written the prescription that works best for me. Ing and Gene and I howl our way through John Cleese in any incarnation.

Even when I'm alone, I'm surrounded by talismans that remind me that I am loved. When I was in the hospital, both my sisters, without consulting with each other, showed up with pieces of my childhood. Sandy brought me a lifelike statue of a turtle. She was delighted when one of the doctors remarked, "Ah, a symbol of longevity," but there was more to the turtle than that. The three of us had always had pet turtles, the little red-eared sliders that, in our youth, were easily purchased in the five-and-dime. We were good at turtle husbandry, so good that when I went off to college, I reluctantly left my by then quite large favorite in the small, tiled lily pond of a friend who promised to overcome her fear of his gaping jaws and feed him off the tip of her finger every day.

Now the turtle Sandy brought me sits under my desk lamp. Our success with turtles was due in large part to our understanding of their need for light, and old habits are hard to break. I often turn the lamp on when I don't really need it, because I sense the turtle's need for drying warmth. Next to the turtle, a carved stone elephant, my gift from Gail, keeps the ties to my childhood strong. When a friend admired it, and I told her it was a get-well present from my sister, my friend's response had a familiar ring. "Oh, neat. Elephants live a long time, right?" And, of course, that's true, but I think Gail's motivation had more to do with childhood prayers.

When I was little, I thought I could not live without an elephant. I wasn't thinking of a baby one. I pictured myself astride a great leathery creature with a high-knobbed skull. I relaxed into the slow, swaying rhythm of our transport, could feel his trunk, warm and bristled with hair, sniffing and blowing into my outstretched palm.

It puzzles me now. I wasn't a stupid child. I surely knew mine was a request not likely to be honored, but my passion was so unrelenting that I forced my father to an empty promise that he would someday get me one. It never happened, and I settled for lots of substitutes. A plush Dumbo who was far more than a toy to me was my constant companion. I insisted that he came to life every night. My stubborn refusal to admit that he was anything but real drove my sisters to distraction and finally forced me to the lie that forever destroyed his power. Sandy and Gail demanded proof that I had been to fairyland with Dumbo. Material proof. Eventually, I went to Woolworth's and purchased two palm-sized china dolls. When I gave these to Sandy and Gail, Sandy pointed out on the top of each doll's head the jagged imprint of the mold that had formed them. "That's from the stem," I told her. "That's the mark from when I picked them from the tree."

Dumbo never again took me to fairyland. And I no longer have my elephant collection, just the recent one from Gail. What happens to those things? Where did that collection go? All the years of holidays when everyone knew the one present sure to please was an elephant in some form or another? To this day, my favorite attraction in any zoo is the elephant house. I love the way it smells, the high ceilings, the dust-filled shafts of light.

Gail gave me something else when I was in the hospital, a silver chain with a pendant bearing a cutout silhouette of the tree of life. "A Quaker cross," she joked as she handed it to me. I put it on and told her I would not take it off until I was healed.

I know that I grant tremendous power to anything in which I can believe. Actively courting the placebo effect, I surround myself with amulets, potions, and chants. These are all things that come to me from friends. Gib, a man I met just briefly at a conference of Georgist economists, hears through the grapevine that I have cancer and sends me a fat packet of articles on meditation and a spiritual approach to healing. It becomes the backbone of my negotiation with this disease. Edie, the closest friend I had when Ingrid and Craig were babies, reappears at just the right moment and sends me a meditation tape (if I had been inclined to push Gib's message aside, this reinforcement brings it home) and a pound of herbal tea reputed to have amazing powers against cancer. I have the luxury of time, and I give myself over to the effort to strike a balance in my life that will make me whole.

July starts out as a good month. I'm feeling pretty strong and happy. When I look in the mirror, I don't see death looking back. It's easy to pretend that nothing has really happened to me. And then one day I'm brushing my hair before climbing in the shower, and I feel a gentle dusting on my shoulders. I look down and discover they are covered with brunette curls. I hadn't planned on going bald. Oh, sure, I had been told that this was likely, but I had decided I wouldn't lose the hair on my head, just on my legs. I am terribly dismayed. It is not a vanity thing. I think some women look really smashing with shaved heads. It is the loss of control that panics me. I had thought I could will my way through this one, make happen what I wanted to happen and hold at bay that which I did not.

Suddenly I'm having a real crisis of faith. All my life, my stubbornness has been my salvation, and now I fear that it has all been a sham. I just pretend I can do anything. I am afraid that I have finally met my match, something more determined than I am. When I asked Dr. Strider why ovarian cancer was such a big killer, he replied, "Because, my dear, it's just like you are, very persistent."

That night when I get into bed, I do something I haven't done since the surgery. I run my hand over my belly, looking for lumps. To my horror, there is one the size of a large orange in the lower right-hand corner of my abdomen. I go limp, feel it is all over with me. This is no nickel-sized tumor. What chance has chemotherapy against something of this magnitude? Gene wants me to call the doctor, but I resist. I'm scheduled in there for a second treatment soon enough. What are they going to do that they aren't already doing? More surgery? And then wait another month till I am healed enough for chemo? No thanks. We knew there were tumors left in there. This doesn't change anything. It makes no difference—only to my sense of hope. I can wait the eleven days until it's time for me to see the doctor.

Erin is my sweetheart. Gene and I are taking her with us to hear the barbershop quartet chorus. Osprey Lakes has a varied summer program in the arts. Tonight's presentation is composed of barbershop quartets from all over this section of Pennsylvania performing together in one huge burst of harmony. We arrive a little late. The show has not yet started, but every seat appears to be filled. Then someone who sees us looking around motions us to the front row. Amazingly, only three seats are left in the house, and they are front row, center. We no sooner sit than the lights dim and the first strains of "When You Were Sweet Sixteen" fill the hall. Erin turns to me, rapt: "Oh, boy, are my mom and dad missing out on something!" I don't think she has been to a live concert before. She has never heard these old songs, they can't possibly call up ghosts from the past for her, can't make her long for an innocence lost, and yet their hold on her is obviously powerful. What meaning can a five-year-old bring to "I love you as I've never loved before—since first I saw you on the village green"?

There is magic in the music and in our shared humanity. The man who wrote this song is dead. The people who first made harmony of its sweet strains are dust, and yet the music reaches across time and generations and holds us in a beat that outlasts the individual pulse and anchors us firmly in the eternal. I cry too easily, I think, always have, so I try now not to cry, but my joy is so intense. I can't take my eyes off the small face beside me, up-turned and bathed in the diffuse glow of the footlights. Its smooth lines and perfect symmetry are an insubstantial thing, the merest flicker in a chain of time. Oh, if I could but stop the race of hours and hold this moment fast. Erin's little mouth is sweetly curved and slightly opened, the lower lip soft and full. Her eyes, just below dark bangs, are wide, the pupils dilated with reflected pleasure.

The song ends and Erin claps with abandon, then waits with fingers lightly poised, almost touching, held just below her chin in hushed anticipation of the next number. She is a happy charmer, her delight so contagious that soon first one and then another of the performers directs his words to her in a sweet intergenerational dialogue of joy. She sits enchanted through one song after another, but shortly after the intermission, I feel a little hand pat me on the knee. I turn to her and she slides effortlessly onto my lap. Resting her head against my shoulder, she falls almost instantly asleep, still smiling, still carried by the music. When it is all over, we wake her up just enough to ride home on Gene's shoulders. The night is very dark and filled with stars. So many stars. Until we moved here, I didn't know the sky could hold so many stars. We walk silently through the streets, the three of us caught in a communion so deep that words would only mar it.

The eleven days are up. It's time once more for my scheduled appointment with the oncologist. Gene drives me to the hospital. I'm eager to see the doctor, want him to tell me this lump is nothing, some postsurgical swelling. I can't wait to get my chemo treatment, want to blast this "postsurgical swelling" into oblivion. Better yet, I want Dr. Silverman to tell me this is all in my head, a figment of my neurotic imagination, or better even still, some-thing I had for breakfast. No such luck. His face reveals nothing. "Umm, yes, I feel it too."

Dr. Strider is on the floor and comes in to check it out. He is incredulous. "I can't believe I would have missed a tumor that size."

I hold my tongue, don't want to remind him how good I am at producing prize-winning tumors, want to believe that nothing deadly happens quite this fast. I have a sudden mental image of myself doing a testimonial-type commercial on TV. I hold a zucchini-shaped tumor the size of a man's forearm aloft. "I rely on Miracle-Gro for all my gardening needs."

Dr. Strider continues with his musings. "This has to be a hydrocele. I did so much work in this area. I wouldn't have missed a tumor this size." He explains that he harvested quite a few lymph nodes from nearby and that it is not uncommon for that kind of activity to cause fluid to accumulate in a saclike growth. They promise to schedule me for a sonogram as soon as possible.

I get dressed and go wait to be called for my chemotherapy. It's not to be. A nurse comes out and explains that my white count is too low for me to go ahead with the scheduled treatment. I had been warned this was the most likely side effect of carboplatin, but I never expected it to happen so early in the process. I am scared and frustrated. Angry. Just when I really wanted something to go after this lump, I am told that I have to wait another week. Dr. Silverman talks to us about Neupogen, a drug that makes white blood cells colonize and increase in number. He recommends that I start giving myself shots in the days following my next chemotherapy treatment, whenever that may be. I don't see how we can afford the cost, over $150 a day. Gene interrupts, "We can't afford not to do it. It won't be forever, just until your treatments are finished."

I can't believe I really need this expensive drug. All my frustration turns to rage, and I go on the attack. I have my first fight with Dr. Silverman. "You're giving me too high a dosage of carboplatin, just reduce the dosage."

He has science and clinical detachment on his side. "There is a strong positive correlation between survival and the strength and frequency of the treatment."

"Well, if frequency matters so much, just reduce the dosage and I'll be able to get my treatments on schedule. I don't like waiting. This thing is just going to keep on growing."

My arguments bounce off him. He is the expert, he's used to comments like mine and is back with an answer without having even to pretend to consider my point. "The strongest correlation is with the strength of the dosage. It's more important than the frequency."

"You don't understand Carberrys," I tell him angrily. "My mother was a Carberry. Carberrys can't take medication. All of us overreact. The amount needed to cure somebody else might be enough to kill a Carberry."

I want Dr. Strider back. He always made me laugh. I can tell that Dr. Silverman is unimpressed with my Carberry argument. I am upset the whole drive home. I feel I've behaved like a fool and have probably made him angry too. I shouldn't have told him the dose was high enough to kill a Carberry. He no doubt thought that sounded like a pretty good idea. I need Dr. Silverman to be on my side. I don't see how he ever can be now. And soon I'm convinced that I've ruined everything.

As soon as we get home, I go upstairs and put my running clothes on. Gene looks a little worried. "Are you sure you're strong enough?"

"I don't care," I snap at him. "If the stupid doctors can't cure me, I'll cure myself. Enough of this passive shit. Waiting to do what I'm told. My body needs to know I have plans for it. I'm not going to just sit around and wait to die."

Oh, God, it feels good to run. I go very slowly, but the Laurel Path lends itself to such a pace. Even at my most fit, I can't run fast on this trail. The footing is too uneven, too many rocks and roots, twists and turns. Chuckles is so happy to have me back, he spins with joy. "Crazy Dog," I call out to him. This is what Gene and I always say when he makes this goofy tail-chasing move. "Crazy Dog!" Thus encouraged, he whirls until he bumps into some rhododendron. Suddenly sober, he collects himself and becomes all dignity as he strides before me. I feel I own my life again. Chemotherapy is not all that stands between me and death. I resolve to meditate regularly, twice a day, no kidding around. And I'm going to drink a quart of the cancer-therapy tea, every day no matter what. I'll go along with Dr. Silverman, do everything he tells me to do. But I'll have my own private plan of attack just in case his lets me down. Running is going to be part of it.

We're into another week and Gene and I are on the way to the hospital for one more stab at respectable white cell counts. But more important for me is the result of the other blood test I had last time we were in. Ovarian cancer produces an enzyme that can be measured in the blood via a test referred to as CA 125. The test they took following my surgery showed a nice drop in the levels, but the results I get today will be the first that show how my tumors have responded to the chemotherapy. On the drive to the hospital, I tell Gene about a new scheme I'm working on. "I get the results of my blood test today. I'm determined my level is going to be below one hundred." Anything below thirty-five is considered normal.

"Don't set yourself up for disappointment," he tells me. "Be satisfied with any drop."

"Nope, I'm not setting easy goals. This is a game I'm going to play, kind of a biofeedback sort of thing. It's going to be below one hundred."

The CA 125 results are great, even better than my most optimistic plans. My reading of forty-seven is so close to normal, I actually begin to feel science is on my side. I'm one of the lucky ones. Not all women have tumors that respond to the drugs. The dice have been tossed, and I've come up with a seven. The white count result is not so good. I'm delayed another week. But this time, I take it more or less in stride. I have my runs. I have my tea. I have my meditation. When I get home, I call Ingrid with the CA 125 result. "We all knew this cancer thing was a mistake," she tells me, and I decide she's right.

Craig and Dee lived with us when they were building their home in Osprey Lakes. One week, Dee and I were grocery shopping. In the middle of aisle three, she excused herself to run to the pharmacy next door. When she returned, I told her she should have made her purchase in the Giant and just thrown it in with the other provisions. "They don't sell home pregnancy kits in the supermarket," she told me, and that's how I got my first glimmer of hope that another grandchild was on the way. I didn't have to wait long to have the promise in that hope confirmed. Craig woke me early the next morning with the good news. "Hey, Mom, it's true, it's true. The test is positive. We're going to have another baby!"

I loved being pregnant when I was expecting my two children, and there is no way to explain the vicarious thrill I got from being part of this little family's expansion. Once the baby began to move, sitting with our hands on Dee's belly became a favored alternative to television for Erin and me. Sonograms were new to me, not a part of the available technology when I had my kids. Craig and Dee were determined not to be told the sex of the little newcomer. Unable to stand the suspense, Erin and I plotted ways to find out. She suggested dressing up as doctors and hiding behind the door of the examining room. If it weren't for her stature, I think that little three-and-a-half-year-old might have had enough moxie to pull it off. As it turned out, we had to stay at home the day of the fateful exam. We thought we'd lost the tell/don't-tell battle to Craig and Dee. We hadn't realized what a powerful ally we would have in as yet unborn, unsexed Kyle.

Craig and Dee came home that night, laughing and excited. Craig leaned over and cupped sweet Erin's face in his hands. "You're gonna have a little brother," he told her. Erin and I seized each other ring-around-the-rosy style and spun about the room chanting the previously agreed upon little-brother name: "David Kyle Fowler. David Kyle Fowler. David Kyle Fowler." She had put in her order for a little sister, but in the triumph of finding out, all that was forgotten.

"What made you decide to let them tell you," I asked.

"Oh, Baboo," exclaimed Dee. "You should have been there! We didn't want to know. We really didn't. But we were watching the sonogram on the TV screen, just a little close-up of the baby's face and shoulders. And then the doctor said, 'Watch, watch. I think this baby is getting ready to suck its thumb.' And, sure enough, Baboo, he opened his mouth real wide and started to move his hand toward his face. But he didn't suck his thumb. He started to wave at us, just like those football players on TV! And he opened and closed his mouth, just like he was saying, 'Hi, Mom!' waving all the while. And I just started bawling and the doctor said, 'Do you want to know the sex?' And, yes, of course we did. Oh, yes, of course we did!"

Suddenly, we knew this little baby. He became real to us that night in a way not possible before. This was a very different thing from feeling him move and kick. He had a face. He had a name. He had a personality. Hi, Mom! The four of us sat around the dining room table and studied the photographs the hospital had sent home with the proud parents. The wave was captured for posterity. It would become the first page of the baby book Dee was already beginning to assemble.

The night before I am due for my sonogram, I have a strange and haunting dream. I'm in the hospital. Doctors and nurses are scurrying all around me, but I am oblivious to them. I've just given birth to the most perfect baby. My delight is so intense. The little fingers peeking out of the swaddling are delicate miniatures, capped with pale pink fingernails, tiny crescent moons. I am given to understand there is medical concern because no one can tell the sex of this baby. However, rather than sharing their dismay, I am puzzled by it. Can't they see the cunning little nose? Don't they know how much I love the wrinkled little brow? When I awake to understand that this was all a dream, I am filled with the deepest sense of loss. My arms are achingly empty. The pain is so acute, it is as if someone had snatched a living, breathing baby from my arms. I feel scooped out, hollow. Absent womb, ovaries, I realize as if for the first time that I will never again have a child, and I am nearly inconsolable. I know it's irrational. After all, I'd already gone through menopause before I had this surgery, but it is as if the hormonal loss had no reality. It took the physical theft of my organs to make me truly barren.

The sonogram itself is almost all that Dee had warned me it would be. I am prepared for the agony of a deliberately generated full bladder. I have an expectation of TV screens, and the technician, perhaps used to sonograms of another type, does not let me down. At my request, she turns the set to face in my direction, explaining as she goes. The "thing," the tumor, the hydrocele, whatever it is, is surprisingly well defined. She taps the TV, her fingernail resting on an undulating octopus of moving filaments. "That's the nucleus." And that's as close to a wave as this disappointed mama is going to get. When I meet with the doctors later, they tell me the test is inconclusive. They can't say that it is a tumor but neither can they say that it is not. A month later, I will have another test, equally inconclusive. They will tell me then that it appears to be somewhat smaller. I will have to take their word for it. When I request TV coverage of the second event, a different technician tells me in a somewhat shocked voice that she couldn't possibly let me see. That kind of information is for doctors only. And suddenly I want Erin, dressed in a white coat with a stethoscope hanging from her neck, hiding behind the examining-room door.

Before I started kindergarten, before formal schooling taught me about gravity and other limits, I was quite certain I could walk on air. The fact that I failed to actually do so I attributed more to a lack of will than to a lack of ability. I frequently stood on the arm of a paint-chipped Adirondack chair and stepped out into space fully expecting to continue uninterrupted on that plane. When I rudely dropped to earth, I always had the same explanation. "That doesn't mean I can't do it. It just means I didn't want to hard enough." The continued challenges of my sisters and peers only served to reinforce my determination. It became such an obsession with me that my parents planned to move me from my third-floor bedroom to one on the second floor. However, they abandoned the idea when they considered that a plunge from two stories would no doubt cause as much damage as one from three. There was no place to house me on the first floor. My attempts at air-walking stopped when I started school, but I have a continued affection for that child who believed she could do anything she really wanted to do.

Chapter 4

August

In August I discover that I can do something almost as transporting as walking on air. I can float on the water like a cork! Swimming has never been a strength with me, so I have not been much troubled by the admonition to stay out of the water until my incision is fully healed. That coupled with the fact that I am supposed to avoid the sun has kept me on the Laurel Path but out of the lake itself. Or it did until a week of August heat, more intense than any of us can remember hitting Osprey Lakes before, finally drives me down to the dock at Edgemere for a quick plunge. I ease myself in cautiously, step by frigid step down the steel ladder at the end of the dock. I take a long pause after each new positioning, waiting for that few inches of leg to become adjusted before venturing any farther. I've never been able to dive, have no desire to learn, much preferring the cold torture of my measured submersion to a nose full of water and stinging belly and thighs. I may be an Aquarian but the water is not my element.

Osprey Lakes has free public transportation during the months of July and August for Lake Association members and their guests. The *Hardly Able* is an old World War I launch boat that has been reconditioned and now carries happy vacationers from the dock at Edgemere across the lake to the beach and back. Ingrid and I secretly call it the *African Queen*, a fantasy helped by the fact that Jimmy Dunham, our launch boat pilot, can, in just the right light, look a bit like Humphrey Bogart. Sometimes when I get tired from taking Chuckles on a walk where his enthusiasm for the next bend in the trail has carried me a bit farther than I had intended, we head for the beach and wait for Jimmy and the *Hardly Able* to give us a lift on the last leg home. Chuckles adores these boat rides. He climbs right up into the prow and poses majestically, head held high, carriage erect, the lake breezes blowing his ears and shiny black coat as we move slowly through the water. Never has there been a more handsome figurehead! No amount of laughter from the bathing-suit-clad children or admiring comment from more formally dressed seniors can break his regal attitude. It is only when the *Hardly Able* docks at Edgemere that he stops being king and becomes just another dog on a walk.

But now I am halfway down the ladder when I see the *Hardly Able* approaching and know that unless I get in quickly, the waves from its churning wake will wash over me with random chill. I drop backward into the water and, to my amazement, immediately bob right back to the surface. I've never been able to float on my back without arching my head and neck until my eyebrows are submerged. And, even then, I've always had to inflate my lungs and madly paddle my arms and legs to keep my nose and mouth above water. But now I find it impossible to sink no matter how hard I try. My entire body floats above the surface of the water. I try every different position I can think of. It doesn't matter what I do. I remain the human cork. Finally, I stretch straight out, folding my hands behind my head as if I were on a chaise lounge. I can lift my head out of the water and stare down at my body, legs, and feet, all well above the surface. I am the unsinkable Heather Remoff! A friend, Dick Deasy, is watching. His wife, Kathleen, will later report his reaction to me. "Dick came home and said, 'Kathleen, you ought to see Heather float.' I nodded my head and said absently, 'Oh, that's nice that Heather can float.' 'No,' Dick told me. 'You don't understand. She doesn't just float. She actually can lie on top of the water.' "

I am euphoric! If only I had understood the system as a child. All my life I've wanted to defy gravity, and now it happens without the slightest effort. The trick is in not trying for control but in just accepting buoyancy when it comes. I shut my eyes. The gentle motion of the water carries me, spins me, sets me adrift. The sun is warm on my body and legs. I am without edges, have no boundaries. Unable to tell where my flesh stops and the water begins, I float free of all moorings. The sun is hot. Am I fire, water, air, or clay? I am all these things and less than any of them. Occasionally, very occasionally, when I meditate, I have this same sensation of losing all definition, of just coming apart into a greater whole. And so it is now. I fall asleep in the water quite easily, thinking, in the moment just before I drift off, what a useful thing this would be in shipwrecks. When I wake, probably only minutes later, I roll over on my stomach and swim, with a grace previously denied me (all I have to do is move my arms), back to the dock.

The rational mind cannot abide mystery. When the initial excitement over my newfound skill wears off, I decide it is all a side effect of chemotherapy. What else could change an absolute sinker into a swimmer almost overnight? I have less body fat than I've had in a long time. Someone suggests that the doctors have removed diseased organs in the same way that one might remove ballast from a ship and with the same effect. However I can't buy that. I don't know about ovaries, uterus, and appendix, but the major and minor omentum are both large fatty structures that cover and protect the intestines. With all that fat gone, I ought to be more dense, not less. In the end, I decide it is my bones, or more precisely, my lack of bone marrow, that accounts for my seaworthy ease in the water. Perhaps I now have hollow bones like a duck and can bob about in joyous imitation of my beloved mergansers.

I'm actually looking forward to my next checkup with Dr. Silverman. After yet another rather heated quarrel between this oncologist and me (he overheard Gene angrily condemn doctors and their games of hide-and-seek and made the mistake of taking me to task for my husband's comment), Dr. Silverman and I have come to a sort of truce. It is not even an armed truce. We are beginning to understand one another. I miss him terribly when he is off at some cancer conference and I have to see someone else. In fact, the worst fight I had with anyone on the medical staff happened when Dr. Silverman was away.

It was the first time I had gone seven weeks between treatments, and I wanted to know what happened to my CA 125 levels when I went that long without chemotherapy. Now it's true, I had had the test three weeks previously, and the results would not have changed a thing as far as whether I got my chemotherapy on that day or not. But I wanted to know simply because

I wanted to know. If my levels stayed constant despite the lack of treatment, it would cause me far less anxiety the next time low white counts postponed the scheduled therapy. Dr. Rudgard, the oncologist who that day deemed my white count sufficiently high to endure another treatment, refused to order the CA 125, even though I pleaded with all the nurses and vowed my willingness to pay the charge myself, on the spot, if need be. I was already hooked up to the equipment, getting prechemo infusions of Ativan, a tranquilizer that I have since learned is not standard procedure for all chemotherapy patients but was considered necessary for emotive me. The thing that infuriates me still is that Dr. Rudgard refused to come talk to me himself about his reasons for not authorizing the test but, instead, sent nurses scurrying back and forth as intermediaries.

My anger and frustration mounted with each refusal. My tears were not of self-pity but of fury at the helplessness of my situation. "The blood is already drawn," I howled. "It's not as if you have to draw more blood. All he has to do is take that little order for lab work and check off one more box!" I kept glancing around the room, hoping to catch the eye of other patients equally tired of doctors making decisions that affected our lives, not theirs. I was sure I could get some kind of rebellion going, a storming of the palace gates, an overthrow, an uprising. Instead, patient after patient averted his or her eyes. It was clear I would get no support. "It's not you I'm mad at," I kept telling whichever nurse carried the latest in the volley of messages between Dr. Rudgard and me. "It's not you I'm mad at!" But they were the ones who were taking my heat. Finally, feeling I had exhausted all my options, I got up out of the reclining chair and pushed my IV pole into the hall.

"Where are you going?" my favorite nurse asked in horror.

"I'm going home." Craig had driven me down that morning. Dee was coming to pick me up in the afternoon. In the irrational zenith of my rage, the lack of transportation was no deterrent. I intended to push my IV pole up Route 42 to Osprey Lakes.

Nurse Nancy rushed to the phone. She was calling the shrink who had been so very helpful in coaching me on how to navigate all the currents and undercurrents of this disease. And suddenly I was broken. There were too many people here I loved. And, of course, there *was* the matter of the thirty-five-mile hike home. I docilely made my way back to my place. (*I* might have considered my behavior docile. The staff had other ideas. One of them later confessed that they had all been impressed by my ability to generate that much fury even as a rather large dose of Ativan was washing through my veins.) I knew then that I had turned some kind of a corner with Dr. Silverman. "This never would have happened if Dr. Silverman had been here," I told Nancy. "He would have ordered the test." And he would have. Scientific curiosity was something Dr. Silverman and I were beginning to have in common.

So now I am eager to get his opinion on the phenomenon of the human cork. I try to couch my question in scientific jargon, talking from my intellect and not my emotions. Even so, when I am finished asking, he begins to laugh. I think we have reached some kind of a middle ground. I am becoming conversant in "medicalese," and he is more comfortable with the idiom of the heart. We are both laughing. "I never heard of such a thing," he tells me. "Perhaps you're learning to levitate. Only you're not very good at it and you need a little help from another medium. The lake acts as your training wheels."

Willis stops by to see me fairly often. Summer is not an easy time for him. Although he loves the work and enjoys long hours on his mower, the "summer people" have little tolerance for his early rising habits. Not a summer goes by without someone appearing at the borough council meeting to protest being awakened at 7:30 A.M. by the snapping of his hedge clippers. Such protest is almost certain guarantee that Willis will thenceforth begin his morning labors at the house next door to the complainant.

When Craig and Dee first arrived in Osprey Lakes, Willis came by to warn Craig of the tribulations of trying to make his living in a July and August community of people who kept late hours. "Summer folks are crazy," Willis warned Craig. "Why, you know that little place over there, back that there road to the beach? No lawn at all. Why it takes me longer to unload my mower than it takes me to cut that grass." Willis pauses here for effect, waits until he is sure we have the setting firmly fixed in our minds. "Well, I was mowing there one morning when the husband comes out and he sez to me, 'Excuse me, but I wonder if you could come back a little later in the day. My wife is sleeping.' " Willis shakes his head, still incredulous at the request.

"Well, I looks at my watch and I sez to him, 'It's nine o'clock. It's *time* for her to be up.' And I kept right on with my mowing. Summer folks are crazy."

If Willis is befuddled by summer people, they are equally confused by him. Those lacking wit make errors of monumental proportions. Why, just last month, one of the renters, angered by Willis's 8:30 A.M. grass-cutting start, made the mistake of charging out of his house, reaching across the mower, turning off the key, and then grabbing Willis himself by the arm and squeezing hard. "It's too early for you to be mowing here," he growled. "I'm warning you. I want you to take your mower and not come back."

Willis was badly shaken by the incident, which occurred the day before the Fourth of July. "I was just trying to git them lawns all nice for their barbecues," he told me in dismay. "I want to tell you, it pretty near ruined my birthday." Willis was born on July fourth. "You know it's not like me to just give up when somebody done somethin' to me. But when that big feller said, 'I'm *warnin'* you,' I was afraid he might go in the house and git a gun and shoot me." Willis is beyond consoling. "If I had a been a younger man, I'd of punched him a good one right in the nose."

Talk about an intrusion into personal space! The story is repeated in hushed disbelief. It is a violation of epic proportions. It is obvious that this city person did not know with whom he was dealing. We are all in awe of Willis's Old Testament approach to justice. He has no tolerance for the urban crimes that get so much press. "Why, them there fellers that rob the 7-Eleven? I'd hang 'em in a tree and let 'em swing and twist until the crows came and pecked their eyes out. And arson fellers? Why, if I seen them, I'd pick 'em right up and throw 'em in their own fire." What is a fitting punishment for someone who interferes with a working man at his work? It is too awful to contemplate but probably falls somewhere between crow-pecked eyes and 7:30 A.M. clippers applied to the immediate neighbor's hedge. Assuming the gentleman in question is foolish enough to return to our mountain next year, we know there will be appropriate retribution. What form will it take? The town has a full twelve months to play with various scenarios. Anyone who doubts that Willis has a loyal army of supporters has only to watch the pleasure with which the imaginary sentences are meted out.

Those with a sense of humor do not necessarily get to sleep later than those who protest Willis's early starts, nor are their peonies guaranteed long life, at least not if they've been foolishly planted in the middle of an otherwise uninterrupted stretch of lawn. However, all is not lost. The flowers may fall, but the town gains another Willis legend with which to liven up the endless round of summer parties. "Willis has done it again," exclaims one good sport with a merry laugh. "I went out and every single one of my lamb's ears was cut off right at the ground. 'Oh, Willis,' I asked him. 'Why did you do that? You've never done that before.' Then he paused and gave me one of those long, steady looks and said, 'Well, I never had a Weedwacker before.' "

This whole "summer people" thing adds an interesting dimension to life in the town. Anyone who isn't at least third-generation born and bred to mountain life is considered a "flatlander." Although Craig works at a laboring trade with all the local folk as peers and companions, I'm afraid that he has been contaminated by my city background and that not even little Kyle, who was conceived and born here, will be considered truly native. "Native" is a distinction to which I aspire.

When I first moved here, a friend and I tried to think of a less judgmental reference than *summer people* versus *local* (with the *yokel* unspoken but too often implied). We finally came up with twelve-month people versus two-month people. However, after spending a winter in Osprey Lakes, I greeted my friend upon her return in July with a discovery. "I know what we should call the local people," I informed her. "Residents." She looked a bit puzzled. I have since heard some of the newer summer people call themselves part-timers and the rest of us full-timers. You'll notice I keep referring to the summer people as "them," trying hard to cast my lot with those with roots. It works only in my head. One of the local residents told me that their name for those who first vacationed here but later retired to full-time residence is "year-round summer people."

Although I will never be local in anyone's eyes but my own, I knew I had crossed the invisible divide when I heard myself explaining to a visiting houseguest the phenomenon of external parasites on domestic pets. She is a dog lover herself and was amazed and impressed that neither Chuckles nor Spike (our much loved, elderly, black-and-white Manx cat) sported a single flea, despite the fact that I am well-known for my refusal to use any kind of chemical pesticide. "Oh," I told her. "We never get fleas in Osprey Lakes until late August. And we probably wouldn't get them at all except that the summer people bring them up."

In the end, it all boils down to something that has more to do with attitude than it does with permanent address or length of time spent on the mountain. Summer people are those who believe Osprey Lakes truly exists only in the months that they are here and that its only purpose is to please them. Summer people assume that roads will not be repaired during July and August, that houses won't get built, and, in fact, usually favor a moratorium on further construction once their own little palace is complete. Summer people believe the world is divided into two classes, those who are on vacation and those who are here to serve them while they are. Summer people protest the cost of public services, without stopping to consider that it is *capacity* they pay for. Our trash collection vehicles and sewage treatment plants must be large enough to serve 3,000 in August. The 123 of us who live here year-round could not possibly need a system that elaborate.

All my local pretensions aside, some of the dearest friends I have ever found live here only a few months a year. Not one of them is a summer person in my eyes. I've never lived anywhere so filled with kindred spirits. Osprey Lakes self-selects for those comfortable with a book or a paintbrush, a hike through the woods. Anyone who wants a pulsing nightlife vacations somewhere else. My friend Bea, who is a poet, lives about a quarter of a mile from me. However, we are both so smitten with the written word that we most often communicate through letters. Bea and I agree that nothing is so restorative as a quiet savoring of the day's mail over a cup of tea. We enjoy communion when we pen our little notes and again when we receive them, but rarely talk face-to-face. Bea has another correspondence going that is far more exotic than the one we share. She and a talented but reclusive poet who lives just a few miles away exchange long and frequent letters. However, they have never met in person and probably never will.

I have more confidence in my running now, and Carol and I have once more taken to the roads. I've promised Dr. Silverman, himself a runner, that I will limit myself to two miles a day, and true to my word, I never go over three. (Not all the oncologists are thrilled with my insistence on running, and this forges a further link in my growing friendship with Dr. Silverman. The first thing he asks me, before he even starts his examination, is, "Are you still running?" and when I assure him that I am, it is as if some affirmation of my ability to withstand the treatments has been given.) Although I run with Carol most of the time, in the week or so following each chemotherapy session, I am too unpredictable and prefer to run alone. On those days, Chuckles and I slowly, ever so slowly, make our way around the Laurel Path.

I may not be feeling terrific on these postchemo runs, but I never fail to be charmed by the lake and its magic. The morning sun is quite lovely. Its reflection bounces off the surface of the water and dapples the undersides of the low-hanging hemlock boughs. It is as if a playful child had cast this sparkling light. My sense of joy is so intense. I feel blessed with a life of ordinary moments holding extraordinary sweetness. I stop just briefly at my spring and touch its waters to my face and tongue, caught in a little ritual that has become a daily pattern on this trail. Perhaps because I am not really watching the placement of my feet as I continue down the path, I trip and begin to fall headlong into some jutting rocks. In a panic, I grab for the closest thing at hand, a thrust of laurel branches, and twist myself into the center of the bush. It is not the soft landing I had envisioned, and I am badly scratched and tangled. The fall has thrown me off-pace, off-balance. Feeling awfully out of kilter, I have trouble getting home and am very glad when the run is over.

A few days later, Craig comes to the door, holding aloft the silver chain and pendant that my sister Gail had given me. "Did you lose this, Mom?"

I reach to my throat in a panic. After all, I had sworn not to remove it until I was healed. Sure enough, my little tree of life is not hanging in its accustomed place. "I must have lost it when I fell. Where did you find it?"

Craig shakes his head. "I didn't find it. I was over by the Outlet Pond, picking up some empty beer cans, when some people in a canoe paddled over, got out, and walked right up to me." Craig looks puzzled. "I have no idea who they were. I've never seen them before. But the woman held up this chain and said to me, 'Look what we found on the Laurel Path.' " He shakes his head again. "I'm pretty sure she thought I was lying, but I said, 'That's my mother's.' She asked me, 'When did she lose it?' and I said, 'I don't know, yesterday?' " By this time Craig has handed the chain to me, and I have already fastened it around my neck. "And then she said, 'Well, we found it Tuesday. It was hanging in a bush.' I reached for it and told her, 'I may be wrong about when she lost it, but I know that's my mother's.' "

I assure Craig that he is right. It is my chain. The only possible answer is that it tangled in the bush and came off when I stumbled. He is relieved that he has not tricked the unknown woman out of her rightful claim. There is something almost frightening about the event. What made those people come show the little silver trinket to Craig? It doesn't look like jewelry of great value. Who were they? Why were they so purposeful in their approach to my son? They couldn't have known that he was my son. They couldn't have known that I had fallen and lost my necklace. Craig and I are too stunned to talk much about the incident, but later that night when Gene arrives from Philly, I share the story with him.

Gene has always had a less fanciful mind than my own, but as we take a late-evening walk around the lake, he allows that there is some mystery here that humbles him. We stand on the footbridge and watch the setting sun. "We are so lucky," he tells me. "There is a magic here."

"Do you think it's a sign?" I ask him. "Do you think it means I will get well?"

He takes my hand. "You don't understand your own magic, do you?" He shakes his head a little bit. "I don't mean to make light of what you're going through, but none of us, none of us who love you, can believe anything except that you will get well. The incident with the necklace is just further confirmation."

Joe the Crow came to us out of the sky. I was eleven at the time, a shy, skinny kid with an unruly mop of tangled curls. My sisters and I liked to sleep late. However, our slothful summer habits came to an end in the two weeks that Joe transformed our lives. One Saturday, Daddy, an early riser with a loud determination to win converts to the cause of daybreak mornings, had given up on the three of us and gone berry picking on his own. We lived in the country, and the acreage around us held a brambled mass of wild blackberry bushes.

By his own telling, Daddy had wedged himself into the center of one such blackberry field and, minus bucket or pail, was picking berries with one hand and piling them into the extended palm of his other. Suddenly, a large crow dropped from the heavens and landed on his outstretched forearm. Joe had arrived.

Joe had a dazzling array of tricks and a quickly established reputation for petty theft. He could bounce a small rubber ball across our stone terrace. He filled an empty Good & Plenty box with pebbles and shook it like a rattle. He would steal any shiny object and fly with it to the top of the walnut tree in our side yard. But, as far as our father was concerned, his best trick of all was his prompt arrival every morning just at dawn. He would land on the porch roof and move between Sandy's bedroom window and mine, pecking on the panes until we got up and came out to play with him. He'd stay for an hour or so and then, seemingly unable to ignore any longer the cawing harassment of the wild crows that circled overhead, would fly off with his companions.

Then one day he just didn't show up, and we never saw him again. It is easy to speculate on Joe's origins as a hand-raised fledgling. His death was at human hands as well. Some weeks later, we learned that a neighboring farmer had been surprised by a "rabid crow" one morning while feeding the chickens. Mr. Jenkins ran for his shotgun, and our dear Joe's life ended in an explosion of black feathers.

Chapter 5

September

September is a lovely month for crows. I'm enchanted by their social habits. "Another crow convention," Gene and I tell each other when we see them gathered along the roadside. Other birds are just now flocking together in practiced synchronized flight, getting ready for the journey south, but crows seem to seek each other's company all year long. And, of course, I see a trace of Joe in each of them. I know what it feels like to have a crow perch on my forearm, the sharpness of the claws, the tentative mass, mass always on the brink of vaporizing with a quick thrust of spread wings. With varnished black feathers, sleek and smooth, a crow has far more substance than actual weight. I love the way a crow hip hops across the ground, the way it turns and cocks its head. Crows see things. Crows have wisdom. Crows break my heart in the same way that September does.

The waxen leaves of the black gum tree are already scarlet. Everything seems poised to vanish. The seasons pass so quickly. All sweetness fades, and yet there is no month more beautiful than blue-sky September. The air is thin and clear. There is a sharpness to my vision. How short the measured cycles of delight. If I would hide from our ephemeral nature, September pulls me back to truth.

I greet the first cold mornings with joy and melancholy. Gene and I now often take Chuckles to the airport for his afternoon walk. The Osprey Lakes airport is an airport in name only. There is no tarmac; no planes land there, or at least they no longer do. This mountaintop sweep of meadow is as lovely a monument to government boondoggle as one is apt to find. In the late forties, the federal government was, as it is now, in the grant-making business. Someone, and here I can only speculate that it must have been a summer person, decided that Osprey Lakes had to have an airport. The rationalization given was no doubt the need for emergency-landing options in a rural county. However, in true emergencies, farmers' fields work just fine, and the only real use the airport ever had was to serve those with their own private planes, hardly descriptive of the local residents of this hardscrabble county.

At one time there was a hangar, but a buried bit of concrete foundation is now the only marker. On the northeast side of the field, just along the edge of the woods, one can find large iron anchor rings embedded in the rock that lies mere inches below the surface of the field at any point. A friend from D.C. calls this "the airport at the top of the world," and there is the sense of being caught at the horizon's curve no matter which pole one chooses to embrace. When at the airport, I always feel cleared for flight, held to the earth by less than gravity.

It is hot here in the summer and very cold in the winter. The airport is a place apart with degrees of climate and vegetation a continent removed from Osprey Lakes, just two miles down the road. The open space is L-shaped, and the far side of the short base is low-growth tundra. Not knowing what to call the plants that dig in here, I have my own names. Reindeer moss. Dwarf blueberry bushes only two inches high and loaded with sweet, dark fruit from July until the first frost. Wild strawberries. Exotic seeded grasses in a range of colors from plum to amber. The mix of wildflowers changes, not by the season but by the day. The rest of the airport is open, blowing meadow. Drifts of flowers splash the field with warm highlights. Violets, daisies, yarrow, thyme, milkweed, and goldenrod each have their hour. The borough mows it twice a year, maintaining its emergency access and holding back the march of blackberry bushes that push in from the edges.

Ingrid loves the airport as much as I do and for all the same reasons. This bone-of-my-bone daughter and I share a heartbeat, and I sense the easy rhythm nowhere more completely than when we are together in the woods and fields. City person though she is, Ingrid has a primal ease in the out-of-doors. She is my gatherer. She knows where the choice wild fungi grow.

Each year we watch our favorite hunting grounds for chanterelles, king boletes, lobster, and oyster mushrooms. The porcini are so plentiful that we dry them to enjoy wild-mushroom risotto even in the off-season. I don't know how it is Ingrid knows the things she knows. Whenever she comes to visit, she goes home with a basket of things from the earth. In the spring, she pulls up the burdock that crowds the roadside. "I'm going to try making pickled burdock root." Stacks of tender leaves from the wild grapevines will travel back to her tiny apartment for blanching and freezing. The next time she comes to us we'll feast on stuffed grape leaves. She treats Sullivan County like a giant grocery store, and we all eat more interesting food as a result.

We begin picking blueberries in July, but the season extends into September. When Ingrid was up last month, she made wild-blueberry jam to share with all of us. Craig, Dee, and the kids helped us pick—everyone but Kyle. His main function was to sit beside the large white enamel kettle into which we all dumped our harvest. Blue face, blue tongue, blue fingers. Even eating with both hands, he was unable to keep pace with the abundance of berries that tumbled into the pot.

The airport is the best place for blueberries. All the local folks who know our love for berry picking promise us that the day will come when we'll work our way around a bush only to find a bear munching on the other side. But although we see lots of bears in Osprey Lakes, we have yet to be surprised by one in berry season. I think we make too much noise, all that laughing and calling back and forth to each other. "You ought to see the size of the berries on this bush!" is answered by "That may be, but the ones over here are really sweet." We each feel that we have found the perfect spot.

The chemotherapy has played some interesting games with my taste buds, but last year when my powers of discrimination were still keen, Ingrid and I could not stop exclaiming over the variations in flavor between one bush and the next. And it's true, no two bushes are the same. Some are obviously different varieties. Bushes growing in identical locations will ripen weeks apart. Even the shapes of the plants range from short and compact to tall with open, reaching branches. The berries on some are almost black and very shiny. Others have skin that is a frosted blue. The seeds can be large enough to crack between one's teeth or so tiny as to be almost nonexistent. But the real difference is in the flavor. Even bushes that look exactly the same bear fruit with contrasting notes. It is more than the difference between sweet and tart. It is an explosion of taste, a smorgasbord of delicious diversity. Wild blueberries forever ruin one for the visually perfect but blandly uniform store-bought variety.

September sun is such a treat, a lovely contrast to the cool air. Ingrid and her friend John are here. She has made a picnic for the four of us. We spread our blanket in the airport meadow and lie back and watch the clouds. It is a child's game. Large billowing white puffs drift and change before our eyes. There are the usual herds of galloping horses, fierce dragons, North Wind faces. By the time one of us draws the attention of the others to the newest magic creature, it has transmuted into something else. While Ingrid unpacks the basket, John runs through the field trailing a stubbornly earthbound kite behind him. We all call out advice. Chuckles bounds along behind John, delighting in this new game. A boy and his dog. Time has such a fluid quality for me now. Past, present, and future shift as easily as the clouds. I see John as a ten-year-old, Chuckles as a pup. In the next instant, I am intensely in the immediate moment, transfixed by the colors and textures of the food Ingrid arranges before us.

Gene and I both love to eat. However, my appetite is fickle now and characterized by cravings more intense than anything I ever experienced during pregnancy. I consume a watermelon a week. As long as something has tomatoes in it or on it, you can get me to go for it. I wake up in the morning wanting V-8 juice. Today, Ingrid plays to my love affair with the tomato, and there is no better month in which to do that than September. As Gene and I watch, she slices local beauties, bursting orbs of firm flesh and shiny seeds. They are deep reddish orange, fading to streaks of gold near the stems. She splits long loaves of crusty Tuscan bread, a treat imported from the city, and layers tomatoes, provolone cheese, basil, and a fragrant mix of olive oil and herbs into majestic sandwiches. She opens a bottle of red wine. (There is sparkling water for me.) "Health-food junk food," Ingrid says as she fills a bowl with crispy chips of dried and seasoned vegetables.

Ingrid has triumphed over chemotherapy's attack on my taste buds. This is the best meal I have eaten in years! Never has food been more savory. It is a moment of perfect happiness. My life now brims with such moments. I can't catalog them all. After we have finished our sandwiches, we gather handfuls of sun-warmed blueberries and pour them over shortbread. The

crowning touch is dripping spoonfuls of Devonshire cream. Feeling nourished, cherished, and content, I rejoice in my family and in the bounty of the
harvest.

So much of my life is consumed now by medical routines. Three days a
week I drive to the hospital for blood tests. I've become a bore on the subject of white cell counts. But at least the fifty-minute drive to Geisinger is
beautiful and restful to my spirit. I feel myself giving up on so much that
matters to me. I'm spending far too much time sleeping, far too little time
writing. I hate poking myself in the belly with Neupogen shots, and even so
it takes forever for my counts to climb enough that I'm cleared for another
treatment. What an optimist I was initially! The treatments were supposed
to be every three weeks. I figured it all out and planned on being finished by
the beginning of October. Now here it is September, and I'm still waiting for
the third of six chemos. Late winter, early spring, is what they're telling me
at this point. I feel as if I'm running a marathon, but in the midst of the
race, some sadistic devil keeps moving the finish line another few miles out.

Dr. Silverman tells me that he's going to switch me from carboplatin to
cisplatin. (The Cytoxan will remain a constant.) Cisplatin is the mean par-
ent of the gentler, sweeter carboplatin. I cry and protest his decision. I know
cisplatin's reputation. Besides, my CA 125s are way down in the normal
range after only two sessions. I'm afraid to trust my life to anything else. Dr.
Silverman prevails. He admits I'll have more nausea but is hoping that cisplatin won't be quite as hard on my bone marrow. "However," he tells me,
"now you *will* lose your hair." My hair is the least of my worries. I've already
lost a tremendous amount, every brunette hair on my head. People think the
shock of this disease has turned me snow-white overnight. But the white hair
was already there, just not as noticeable when mixed with darker companions.
I rather like the white look and have taken to calling myself a geriatric
blonde. When I was a teenager, I had friends who bleached their hair almost
this pale. Platinum blond, they called it. How appropriate, as carboplatin
and cisplatin both use platinum as a base. I who own so little jewelry am suddenly awash in precious metals. The million-dollar baby. The question re-

mains: Do blondes really have more fun? It doesn't feel that way to me. When I'm in a less playful, more philosophic mood, I refer to this new silver coif as my enlightenment hair.

I bump into Dr. Strider in the lobby on my way out. Crying on his shoulder, I voice all my fears about the proposed switch. "Come on," he tells me. "Not to worry. Cisplatin is the gold standard by which carboplatin is judged." As always, he makes me feel better, and I drive home smiling.

Eventually I get the treatment, and I do feel sicker than I thought it possible to feel. The good news is that my CA 125 stays low. The bad news is that the white counts prove as vulnerable as ever. But the decision has been made. Everyone agrees. I'll stay with cisplatin. The fight has turned ugly now. The stakes are high. Well, I think I'm ready. Let the games begin. I'll do whatever it takes to beat this bastard cancer.

It has been years since I've enjoyed red meat. The literature that the hospital gave me when I was first diagnosed warned that meat might taste bitter while I was undergoing chemotherapy. This was of no concern to me. It was rather like asking a child to give up spinach for Lent, and I made no attempt to even taste a hamburger. Now, however, cisplatin has turned me into a carnivore. I crave steak with a vengeance. Gene is delighted. We've always been on different dietary wavelengths, and this new meat-and-potatoes me is a creature he loves to indulge. He has taken over most of the cooking. So little looks appetizing to me in grocery stores that I can spend an entire hour in one and come out with nothing but laundry supplies. Gene broils steak every weekend, and I tear into it like a 1950s football player.

With the craving for steak comes a craving for Reuben sandwiches. When Gene goes back to Philadelphia, Craig and Dee take over the challenge of feeding me. Craig puts together a really mean Reuben, and I get door-to-door delivery service. (Carol's husband, Bill, makes an equally good sandwich. I find myself happily spoiled on several fronts.) What a strange thing this is. Suddenly I don't care if I never see another lentil or warm white-bean salad. Tomatoes are still a hit, however, and when not cooking steaks, Gene takes me down to the Barn for a spaghetti dinner.

The Barn is our local bar, located just a mile or two outside of town.

There is a restaurant in back that gets quite a bit of play during July and August (their red sauce is really good), but it doesn't matter how many summer people eat there; the Barn belongs to those who live here year-round. All you have to do is come in through the bar entrance and you know you are among those who call the place home. The barstools are almost always full. Those with urban sensibilities hesitate at the door, fairly certain that the directions they've followed are not the directions that were given. The owner barely looks up from stacking glasses: "Restaurant's in the back." I don't know that the people in the front, at the bar, ever eat, but it's obvious that they drink. By dinnertime, several of them, predictably the same several, are already pretty well seasoned.

The room is dim, smoky, relaxed. Everyone is leaning on the bar, and only familiarity with individual habits enables one to tell at a quick glance who is propped up because he needs to be and who is simply comfortable. A pool table and pinball machines are off to one side. The place is especially formidable late at night. I've never been there in the midnight hours, but once Ingrid had a friend visiting from Manhattan who, unaware of Sullivan County's lack of late-night business activity, was forced to the Barn's cigarette machine shortly before closing time. Ingrid waited in the car while he ran in. Tony, who is of Asian ancestry, came out terrified. "I was sure someone was going to start having Vietnam flashbacks!"

My favorite Barn story happened in the off-season. The restaurant in back is actually quite nice: clean, bright, a good place to bring the family. A stuffed grizzly bear with a fish in his mouth stands in one corner. Heads of his black bear cousins hang on the walls. It was early spring and a friend whose wife had been called back to the city was dining alone. Shellie, his waitress, is a young local woman with a small daughter. Since Bob was the only customer for dinner, Shellie was easily able to handle her divided duty as bartender/waitress. The kitchen has a door that opens into the dining room and another that leads into the bar. When Bob inquired about Shellie's little girl, Samantha, he learned that it was her birthday. Shellie was planning to take advantage of the light dinner crowd and bake her a cake while on duty. Bob was halfway through his linguini when he heard Shellie head into the bar and ask of those propped on the counter, "Okay. Who wants to lick the bowl?"

September draws to a close, and I feel caught with the same bittersweet melancholy with which I began the month. Does nothing last? Are all seasons so fleeting? And then I remember that just after I'd finished writing my memories of Joe, the black-magic bird of my youth, I came out of our house for my morning run with Carol only to find a large crow feather by the front gate. Obsessed with signs and portents, I decide that the placement of the ebony feather was no casual thing, but a reminder that nothing really vanishes.

My father was always a man of outsize dreams and instant enthusiasms. The slightly shabby gentleman's farm that we were renting when Joe found us seemed to intensify this already existing trait. Daddy was reared on a working farm. He should have known that his dream of ten acres and independence was hopelessly romantic and doomed to fail. However, he had accomplices in his mission. Sandy, Gail, and I fell into the whole project with an eagerness that matched his own. We hadn't yet grasped our father's problem with follow-through.

We quickly filled the barn with chickens, ducks, pigs, a pony, and rabbits (in exponentially expanding numbers). Mother, the one realist in the family, pointed out the lack of running water in the barn and its distance from the house. We ignored her and bought the foundation stock for a flock of sheep. And every morning after driving her husband to the train that took him to the city advertising agency where he worked, Mother came home and carried water to all the waiting critters in the barn. Her daughters, I am ashamed to admit, never managed to get out of bed in time both to water the animals and catch the school bus.

Mother put her foot down when Daddy sent away for literature on goat dairies. "No goats," she said. Daddy waited until her birthday and then gave her a Nubian-cross doe with two cunning kids poised by her flanks. It was the beginning of the end. Those kids had springs in their feet and mischief in their hearts. No fence could contain them, and in their search for the perfect sliding board, their sharp little hooves ruined not only our car, but the cars of any persons foolish enough to pay us a visit. Mrs. Hupp, the mother goat, inspired by an erratic milking schedule, learned to tuck her head under her hind leg and drain her own udder. The last straw came when a laughing 4-H leader informed Daddy that the two kids, rather than being nannies, were hermaphrodites (a condition common in goats) and useless as future milk producers. The goats were sold, and one by one, our dreams fell away.

Chapter 6

October

I am my father's daughter. Open any closet in our house and you will find evidence of abandoned dreams. Years ago, I came home from the summer Olympics in Montreal with a half dozen field hockey sticks and the address of a field hockey club in our area. I was certain my family and I would rise to fame for our skills in ball-handling. We never went to a single meeting of the club. For one brief season I attended every Irish festival within a day's drive, and my file cabinet still has all the information on bagpipe and step-dancing lessons. I step-dance only when asleep. Soon after we purchased Chuckles, my library expanded to include four volumes on training gun dogs. I am terrified of guns and wouldn't have one in the house. Chuckles' tracking leads were used only twice. They hang beside dear deceased Scoobie's old pulling harness. Scoobie did sprint across the frozen lake dragging me on a sled, but we somehow missed the Iditarod. Half-finished manuscripts gather dust under the bed. I go into everything with such enthusiasm and then grow quickly bored when real discipline and commitment are required. Will it be the same with this fight against cancer? Now that the battle is getting hard, will I step out of the ring before the final bell? I have certainly begun a campaign in that direction.

The thing is this: I don't know which is worse, the treatment or the disease. I never counted on feeling quite this sick. Do they really have to come so close to killing me to find a cure? How do they know I'm not cured already? I want so much to quit, but I don't trust my own judgment. What I really want is for some medical expert, someone in a position of authority, to tell me that I've had enough, that it's okay to walk away from cisplatin. So I'm playing a new game with new rules: I will follow all my doctor's orders to the letter, but I am allowed to marshal every debating skill that I possess in an effort to get him to change those orders. I'll quit chemotherapy only when Dr. Silverman tells me I can, but he is going to hear about every negative impact of this treatment.

Therefore, I am delighted one morning in October when the world fractures before me. Carol and I have just finished our morning run. She has headed back to her house, and I am cutting across the village green with the intent of letting Chuckles run home on the Laurel Path. Suddenly, everything around me is broken. Nothing in my entire visual field makes sense. It's as if reflected reality were painted on a mirror, only someone has dropped the mirror and broken it into hundreds of thousands of pieces. Tiny disconnected shards float at varying distances from me. Unable to tell where the ground is located, I freeze and watch while bits of the world move first toward me and then away. The pieces are so small and so inconsistent in location that they cannot be put together jigsaw-puzzle fashion. The entire episode probably lasts less than five minutes, but it feels like forever before the fragments begin to sort themselves into increasingly larger wholes. At last I am able to see two dogs, both of them Chuckles, running toward me. This visual sleight of hand is good; it is impossible for me to tell which is the real Chuckles and which is his refracted double. By the time he presses against me, they have merged into one and my world is whole and familiar once more.

"Okay," I think triumphantly. "This is it. This is the end of cisplatin!" I can't wait to get home and call Dr. Silverman.

His response is not what I had expected. "Let me call you right back. We'll bring you in sometime today for an MRI of your brain."

I interrupt, "There's no way I have a brain tumor." Dr. Silverman was obviously not around when I declared my brain off-limits.

He continues, "It's better to catch these things early. I'll call you right back and let you know what time we have you scheduled."

I am indignant. "I know I don't have a brain tumor. You're just wasting our health-care dollars! This is the cisplatin that's doing this."

Do I let Dr. Silverman win these arguments in the same way that I let young children beat me in Parcheesi? All I know is that I sit by the phone and wait for his call and don't argue with his advice not to drive in case the episode recurs. Carol is my chauffeur and nurse, even sitting beside me while I lie in the missilelike MRI chamber. I'm not afraid. I seem unable to believe that this thing has touched my brain. The photo images prove me right. And it is while looking at the films that I am glad I consented to the procedure. Dr. Silverman makes the inevitable joke about being surprised to find I have a normal brain, but he is obviously proud of the current technology. "We didn't used to be able to get pictures like this without a saw." It is truly amazing, looking into my own brain. However, I am a little disappointed, not in the quality of the prints, but in what they reveal. I remember hearing in high school biology that the more wrinkles on the surface, the greater the intelligence. I wish for more and deeper fissures but leave that observation unspoken.

So what has caused my fractured vision? No one will allow that it could be cisplatin. All a battery of tests can turn up is a blood sugar reading in the low forties. I've never had low blood sugar in my life and try to lay the blame for that solidly on my chemical nemesis, but I can't get anyone to buy my argument. "Make sure you eat something before you run" is the advice from the endocrinologist. Can it really be that simple? Nothing more than an empty stomach?

I love October in Osprey Lakes. Everyone goes home. The water gets turned off on the fifteenth of the month, and since most of the summer people rely on the Water Company for their supply, they flee the mountain. Those of us with wells are smugly self-sufficient, not afraid of winter, here for the long haul. I remember my first autumn in Osprey Lakes. Scoobie, the Lab/husky/mystery mix that was our dog then, was helping me haul leaves down the hill behind our house and into a compost pile in the woods. I would rake the fallen beauties into the center of a tarp, and Scoobie and I would each grab a corner and pull. As soon as I dumped the leaves, that determinedly helpful dog would take the empty tarp in his mouth and race back up the hill with it all by himself. He wouldn't put it down until he was beside the next raked pile.

We tell people that Scoobie was the smartest dog we have ever encountered, but perhaps that assessment does a disservice to Chuckles. Scoobie put his intelligence to work doing for us. Chuckles works to please himself. Here is the contrast. Scoobie started life as a city dog and, in true urban fashion, accompanied me on my weekly walks to the grocery store. From the time he was about six months old, he insisted on carrying the groceries home for me. In the beginning, his determination was more of a nuisance than a help. He would leap up and just grab packages out of my hand, often ripping them in the process. One day, when the bundle I carried was a small one, I got disgusted and just shoved it at him. "Here! You want it so much, you carry it!" He did, and from then on we were a shopping team. Once I learned to accommodate his desire to help, his habit really was useful. At the supermarket, I would get one large brown paper bag and fill it with light items, leaving just enough room to fold the edges over so that he could get a good grip on it. I'd walk home with his lead looped over my wrist and a bag of groceries tucked under each arm. Scoobie would prance along, head held high so that his bag wouldn't drag on the ground. Drivers would pull over and yell out the car window, "How did you ever teach him to do that?" There was no way to explain. My animals always teach me more than I teach them. Old Scoob wouldn't put his bag down until he deposited it squarely in the middle of the kitchen floor.

Now Chuckles is another matter. One of the early rules of the house was that he was not allowed to get up on the furniture. And he didn't. He didn't need to. When seeking a comfortable nap, he would pull the cushions off the couch and curl up on them on the floor. He respected the stated limits but still got what he wanted. He has never helped me rake leaves, but he has given me lots of laughs with his clownish ability to serve his own ends and still stay within the letter of the law.

But to get back to that warm October day when Scoobie and I were working in the yard; I was just tidying up the last few leaves along the edges of the slate sidewalk in front of our house when I heard the most musical sound coming from under my feet. Scoobie pulled up short and stood with one ear cocked toward the ground. Somewhere below us the earth was singing. It was a water sound but a deep water sound, not the light, happy notes of a splashing brook. This was joy in a minor key with the hollow echo of impending loss. I stood enchanted, puzzled by the source of the gurgling subterranean melody. Only later did I learn what had cast this spell. Mark Houst, our third-generation plumber, overheard me describing the phenomenon to someone in the post office and interrupted with the rational answer: "I turned the town water off today. You heard the water leaving the pipes."

The post office in Osprey Lakes is the village center. Although the town is tiny, there is no house-to-house delivery. If you want your mail, you have to go to the post office to pick it up. Frank Miller, our postmaster and deputy game warden, knows more than he tells. He doesn't have to read anybody's postcards. All he has to do is listen when people come to collect their mail. Frank reliably has it sorted and in the boxes by 10 A.M. I've always said that, in Osprey Lakes, you can have a social life without ever having to give a party. All you need do is head to the post office at ten in the morning. Everybody is there. It's more entertaining than any electronic bulletin board and requires no special equipment or technological skill.

In addition to the word-of-mouth relay of information, there is a huge corkboard in the vestibule. In the summer months, the notices are layered and overlapped. It would take the good part of a morning to read them all. The summer kids are an entrepreneurial lot. Budding bike and in-line-skate repairmen post their hours. There are offers to baby-sit, dog-walk, or bake the cake of your dreams. Willis has a lock on the lawn-mowing business, so there are no advertisements for work of that sort. Not all of the flyers are economic in nature. There are typed schedules of summer activities: plays, concerts, bird walks, star-gazing, swimming lessons, acting workshops, hikes, and bike rides.

In October, the bulletin board gets a clean-slate start. Every year, the same photocopied cartoon mysteriously appears. A woman is lifting the slanted, outside cellar door and calling into the basement, "Okay, you can come out now. The summer people have gone." One of the first off-season notices to go up is the sign-up sheet for the dollar spaghetti dinner sponsored by the Civic Club. When I want my city friends to know how far back in time I have moved, I find opportunity to slip casually into the phone conversation the fact that I must hang up and get myself to the one-dollar spaghetti dinner. Most of the town's 123 residents show up hungry and leave happy, full of spaghetti, meatballs, tossed salad, garlic bread, beverage, homemade cookies, brownies, cakes, and pies. The event is obviously not a fund-raiser. It is a reinforcement and celebration of community. The intent is that attendance be limited to those who live here. However, the year we put in a new sewer system, the supervising engineer was in town the night of the spaghetti dinner, and the borough secretary invited him to attend. She was perfectly willing to pay for his supper, but he absolutely refused her generosity. He couldn't wait to submit the cost of his evening meal on his expense report.

I know that by the end of October, almost every leaf will be gone. And so, even though I'm very tired, Chuckles and I wander a bit far afield on our afternoon walks, exploring new territory. I am often deliciously possessed. There is a sense of floating through the woods. I seem to be riding life with such a loose rein that sometimes I turn and look behind me, checking to make sure I'm still leaving footprints.

Every now and then I hear music, but it is not the stuff of heavenly choirs. My tune of choice is tinkling whiskey piano, Tom Waits sort of stuff. How can someone who has never frequented bars be so drawn to the ache of lonely, smoke-filled roadhouses? I don't know the song but the melody will not leave me. This refrain has a merry, music-box quality, but it is a music box in a Bushmills bottle. The tune may be lighthearted, but I sense the lyrics hold the darker truth of heartbreak. Even so, I am drawn into the dance.

My imaginary twirls lift me several feet above the ground. This is not a thing of the body. I've learned to let go of that. I suppose if someone came upon me in the woods, they would see that physical self just standing there, but the me that matters, the me that dances, is high in the air, spinning in time to the music. And when the music dies and I pause briefly and look down at the grassy place where I had been standing, it is just as I had feared it would be. There is no worn spot to mark my passage. It is just as I had suspected. There is not a single trace of all that joy.

I am counting on the usual delays in my chemotherapy treatments, and I am not disappointed. I wanted to wait until after Grace's Run to be zapped, and

I will get my wish. Grace Andrews was a remarkable native of Osprey Lakes whom I know only by reputation. She raised fourteen children and then started her own college education. Grace took up running at about the same time. While on a five-mile run that included a lap around the lake, she was struck and killed by a hit-and-run driver. Every year her children return to Osprey Lakes to hold a three-and-a-half-mile road race in her memory and honor. The Grace's Run Memorial Trophy is engraved with the name of the first female over fifty to cross the finish line each year. When we were new residents here, I once managed to accomplish that. The next year, the woman who won left me in her dust at the starting line, and I never saw so much as her back the entire rest of the race. I have no illusions about my performance in this October's event, but I am determined to compete in the race. My stated goal is simply to finish.

Race day dawns clear and shining, October at its best. We have a lot of sugar and red maple in Sullivan County, and these blaze in shades of orange and scarlet. Although they tell me a blight will eventually kill all the beech, there are still enough of them to mass the woods with gold. Dark hemlock is the counterpoint in any season, but the contrast is most vivid in the fall. The sun is so bright I worry I'll be too hot and whine that it would be better to have rain.

I'm not usually one to fuss about the weather. It's just a case of nerves. The last time I ran more than two and a half miles was six months ago. I get tired just sitting in a chair. What makes me think that I can do this? Besides, I know myself. How is Miss Competitive Spirit going to be able to endure running dead last? It used to kill me in a race to be passed by someone wearing mascara and elaborately styled hair. Now I worry that I may *actually* kill myself pushing too hard not to be passed by the overweight and infirm. I *am* the infirm. What kind of cruel trick is this? Pride goeth before a fall. I think I had this one coming.

Gene has not run in months. He offers to run with me. We've never done this in a race. Not even in the 10K we ran on our honeymoon did we run together. Gene was always out in front. I try to turn down his offer to serve as my governor. He thinks I'm being noble. I keep the truth to myself. Incredible as it may seem, I fear that he's in worse shape than I am and will hold me back. In true Walter Mitty fashion, I harbor secret fantasies that the old killer instinct will lift me above the limitations imposed by low blood counts, and I will surprise us all. Gene, however, is insistent and I finally relent. If I don't do well, I'll use him as my excuse.

I know in the first half mile that I'm in trouble. Oh, it's nothing dramatic and life-threatening, but it's clear that although I didn't really mean it when I told people that my intent was to run in the back, my body thought that sounded like a splendid idea. We are dead last at the first mile marker. By the halfway mark, even the sag wagon and ambulance have passed us. We can no longer see the rest of the race. Gene is breathing hard, but it's clear that he could run faster than I am going. Suddenly I'm very grateful for his presence. It would be awfully lonely back here by myself. And finally, with no other choice before me, I give up and do what I said I would—I pace myself to finish and take pleasure in the golden drifting leaves, the race, the good man beside me.

I assume that the finish line will be deserted by the time we get there, but I could not be more wrong. People are yelling out encouragement, cheering me on. Those from out of town must be perplexed. I doubt that even he who won the race got a more enthusiastic reception. Familiar faces from town crowd into a corridor as Gene and I head for the finish, hand in hand, a deliberate tie for last.

As soon as I stop running, I feel immediately chilled and hurry home to a hot shower. Gene will hang around and watch the awards ceremony. I'm just pulling on dry clothes when I hear Gene, breathless and excited, banging on the bathroom door. "Hurry up! You won the Grace Andrews trophy! You have to get back for the awards ceremony."

It's unbelievable but true. I was the *only* woman over fifty in this year's race. The photographer from the *Sullivan County Review* is waiting when I get back. Gene and I love this loopy, local paper. We joke that it's impossible to get your picture on the front page unless you are either a dead animal or are holding one. (Hunting season is big up here. Dead turkeys, deer, and bears get top billing.) That is, of course, a bit of an exaggeration. Litters of puppies and pastoral scenes of cows grazing in shaded pastures are also pretty standard stuff. At any rate, I laugh through my tears as Doc Shoemaker, local veterinarian and owner/editor/photographer for the paper, snaps my picture. I know this isn't front-page stuff, but it's a thrill anyway. After the race, the Sweet Shop gives ice cream cones in exchange for race numbers to all competitors. The day is grand, both in the living and in the memory. Later, the "Sully" will arrive scattered through with dozens of photos of the race, mine among them. (I will clip out the picture and send it to Dr. Silverman and the oncology staff at Geisinger.) Competitive to the end, my only disappointment is that they include my "winning" time. Don't they understand? Some things are better left unsaid.

By the end of the month, it has turned suddenly cold, and Dee and I fear the ground will freeze before we get in the daffodil bulbs we ordered in a burst of summer enthusiasm. Three hundred bulbs! Were we out of our minds? Gene and Craig rise to the occasion, and the six of us (Erin and Kyle insist on helping too) spend most of one weekend fighting rocks. Not one bulb goes in without a struggle. How do trees manage to grow here? I fear we've killed every potential daffodil. Besides waiting until too late to plant, the recommended six- to eight-inch depth has proved impossible. By late Sunday afternoon, the job is finished, but I feel more disheartened than triumphant.

Even when working in the best of conditions, I am a bulb-planting skeptic. How can something so dry and brown endure through winter's cold and still produce such thrusting, bursting life at the first hint of the sun's warmth? Life's miracle is nowhere more neatly summarized for me than in the waving first blooms of early spring. I've never understood the fury that supposedly accompanied publication of Darwin's *Origin of Species*. How could anyone protest being placed in nature's camp? I find my salvation there. Descended from angels? Held apart from life's ebb and flow? Why do we want to claim some artificial immortality? It is *mortality* that defines life as we know it. Death and renewal. Right here before our eyes, not in some far-off, exclusionary club. What could be more beautiful than the turn of seasons? Who could ask for more than inclusion in that process?

In the physical exam that precedes my fourth chemotherapy treatment, Dr. Silverman presses deep in my belly and makes an encouraging observation: "That mass seems to be shrinking."

"Of course, it is," I answer quickly. "I've been drinking red-clover-blossom tea."

He doesn't respond to that at all. No change of expression crosses his face. It is only later, probably under the influence of Ativan, that I reflect on what I've done and feel deep regret. How could I so blithely dismiss his skill and efforts? Do Cytoxan, carboplatin, and cisplatin get no credit at all? And what about the doctor who has devoted years of his life to research and training? I know he has given lots of time and thought to finding just the perfect balance. In my clumsy attempt to claim credibility for my alternative but complementary approach to healing, I fear that I have been unkind. I should apologize, but I don't see Dr. Silverman again that day, and by the next time that I do, I want nothing more than to forget the whole incident.

I've stopped hating doctors, but in the two weeks following this treatment, I am so truly, horribly sick that I am no longer sure I want to give cisplatin credit for anything at all. *I* may not hate doctors, but I seek out my friends who do. I plead with every one of them for permission to cancel this whole thing. I call all the people who love me but have reservations about the medical profession, hardly a random sample. And even with that research bias, to a person they urge me to follow doctor's orders. They fear the disease more than I hate the treatment. "You have to do it," one friend firmly tells me. "You have too much invested in suffering to quit now." But it is Ingrid who finally convinces me to give up this campaign to terminate the chemotherapy. No one loves me more than she does. She has felt my pain with an intensity equal to my own. (There are drawbacks to shared-heartbeat love.) She tries to come up from the city to help me through the days following each treatment. She has known my agony firsthand. And she responds with near terror when I talk about stopping. It works—every maternal instinct in me wants to protect her from the source of her fears. I resign myself to hanging in there. Everything passes, and this will too. A month that has begun with the fear that I possess a congenital inability to finish anything ends with a resolution to break with family tradition. I'm not giving up until I get the recommended six treatments.

From the time I was a young teenager, I pictured myself a November bride. My friends borrowed wedding magazines from older sisters and swooned over white tulle and lace, billowing clouds of silk organza tucked and stitched with tiny seed pearls. There were veils and trains, pink roses, baby's breath, and small pale lilies. Everything was light and airy with romance and June.

My dreams had a more somber tone. Instead of a wedding gown, I wore a floor-length, gored, gray woolen skirt. I suspect I was unduly influenced by a Gibson Girl print that hung over my mother's bed, because I saw a high-necked white blouse with leg-of-mutton sleeves and a single red rose at the throat. The setting was desolate, somewhere cold, for snow piled up outside the small log cabin where I felt the ceremony would take place. The groom was a mere faceless sketch of some outdoor type. Only a half dozen close family members were there. No minister that I could see. The clearest image was the fire, and it burned and danced above a banked bed of molten coals glowing with pulsing heat and holding a winter's worth of flame.

I guess I knew that some things weren't real, for I never told either of my husbands of my vision, and there was no attempt to set a November date. May and September were our months of choice. I no longer sense prophecy in that dream. I understand now that it was nothing meant to happen, but symbolized, instead, something that already had. Perhaps Dave, my first husband, and Gene should have been warned that I would never make a lighthearted bride, for I was already wed to something darker.

Chapter 7

November

November has always been my favorite month. I have spent much of my life nursing a stained melancholy, not black despair but a state nonetheless tinged with dark-edged sorrow. Winter has always suited my veiled moodiness. I have found strange comfort in the cold. There is no demand for bright laughter. Simple endurance is all that is required. Winter is a waiting game, and in the cold months I have found the quiet patience of a cat.

We have true winter in Osprey Lakes. The snow begins early and, in a good year, piles steadily deeper through all the dark months. The lake freezes sometime after Thanksgiving, and we are locked into a stillness that takes the breath more than does the cold. I have always explained my affection for this frozen landscape by reference to cross-country skiing, ice-skating, weekend camaraderie with friends in front of a wood-burning fireplace. And, certainly, the pleasure I take from all these things is accurate, but the truth is deeper and less accessible even to those who love me.

However, this year, this cancer year, has robbed me of the satisfaction I once found in my well of sorrow. I still love the gray cold, the sense of isolation, but depression has lost its hold on me. I no longer turn inward to gnaw on my own heart. I am startled to realize that although I often have been angry, sick, weak, and frustrated in the past seven months, I have not once been depressed. Where is the weighted lethargy that, in the past, has pinned me to my chair, overwhelmed by the lack of purpose in the numbing wall of tasks that faced me?

I seem cured of a lifelong affliction. Can it be that my blue moods masked a fear of death? I have always claimed, rather too quickly I see now, to be comfortable with the thought of dying. This year I've learned that I have lied to myself and others. I was terrified of the loss of self that seems to accompany life's end. But now, I have a different understanding and actually see ego as more of a burden than a gift. It is the source of almost all our pain. Individual identity is an isolating, striving thing and offers little comfort.

There remains the matter of the unknown. It is certainly hard to leave that which I love for that which is all uncharted with no turning back should the promises prove false. I am not eager to die, but neither am I afraid of it. Death and I are on better terms now. I know his bony, hollow face and find a certain beauty there. When all that is false and insubstantial is stripped away, there is only the purity of weathered truth.

Muncy Valley follows the creek that traces its way around the bottom of our mountain. It is folded in between the soft hills that pass for peaks in this part of the country. Much as I hate to leave Osprey Lakes for any reason, this narrow glen is uncommonly beautiful, especially so in November. For its entire length Muncy Valley is never more than one farm wide. One of these plots, the Frazier place, is a working farm, neat and no-nonsense. Its house and barns boast clean, functional lines. In the green bounty of summer, tall stands of corn almost hide the outbuildings, positioned as they are far from the road and close to the creek that, from this vantage point, is invisible in any season. Although one can't see the water, its passage can be marked by the tall trees and waving vegetation that line its banks.

When November comes, the corn stalks are all laid low, pale silvered tan, pithy at the core, any lost ears fair game for deer and crows. Now the trees along the creek's edge are what draw and hold me. When all was green, I missed their essential nature. Sycamores, too leathery of leaf, are not much loved by me in summer, but when the gray quiet of impending winter strips them bare, they rise with haunting beauty in the fading light. The rough, mottled bark of July falls as surely as their leaves, exposing the loveliness of bleached and skeletal remains. There is a graceful sadness in the sycamore trees. They gleam like polished bone. Like my bones. Like your bones. Like the bones of us all.

Willis has a Muncy Valley address, although he actually lives away from the valley up on Beaver Lake Road. The Myers family is a prolific one, scattered throughout these parts, all of them as simple, unassuming, and hardworking as their name. I don't think I'm exaggerating when I say that Willis's nephew Chet is the best mechanic in the world. His garage is near the point where Myers and Beaver Lake Roads meet. It's as rural an area as one could find, the spartan brown frame structure the only commercial activity in sight. The earliest part of the garage was built in 1920, the new wing added in the forties. When I was first inquiring after a mechanic and Carol's husband told me where to find Chet, I protested that the building was no longer in use. Bill laughed. "It just looks that way. The only light Chet ever has on is the one above the spot where he is working."

Chet is as careful with my money as he is with his own. With cars as with buildings, his philosophy seems to be to fix nothing that isn't broken. As a result, driving up to the garage is like driving into history. The inside is even more wonderful than the out. Ancient wood and glass candy counters line the office walls. There are old calendars, photographs of record snowstorms. The mechanic's area has diagonally placed, wooden floorboards that are clean and tidy but well oiled with years of service. I drive a 1983 Toyota Tercel, and although I love it dearly, my affection does not extend to keeping it clean. I am always shamefaced when I bring it down to Chet and worry that he may feel the need to sweep it off before he is willing to drive it into his spick-and-span work area. I have to admit that my aging car is an embarrassment to my husband, who probably wishes Chet were less talented at keeping it on the road. Our house does not have off-the-street parking, and Sullivan County's heavy winters, complete with various snow-melting chemicals, have the car well pockmarked with rust. Chet's son, David, with skills worthy of the Myers name, has kept the hatchback door inspection-worthy by welding replacement metal pieces to it. Gene prays for the day when the car won't start, but I don't think Chet is going to let that happen.

Chet's bills are themselves a work of art, so much so that I have never thrown one out. I'm certain he never got less than an A in penmanship. Every single item that has gone into a repair is individually listed with the price.

"Nut 4¢. Bolt 8¢. Vacuum Hose 15¢." If he uses a third of a quart of washer fluid, he charges you for just a third. One item did have me confused, but I didn't want to ask Chet for fear of appearing to challenge the billing system. Sometimes he charges me for the cost involved in getting a part and sometimes he does not. Even when he does, the charge is never the same—$3.75 one month, $2.55 another. I asked Bill Feese what was going on. I knew there was nowhere Chet could drive for parts without its involving at least an hour's trip. His bills could not possibly reflect labor costs. "Oh," Bill told me. "That one is easy. He doesn't charge to get parts if it's an item he has in stock. When he has to go get parts, he divides the cost of the drive equally among the number of customers who need something from that trip." For the first time in my life, I don't have to try to protect myself from mechanics who might take advantage of my lack of automotive knowledge. I love dropping the car off and telling Chet, "Just go ahead and repair or replace anything you see that needs it."

It has been a good year for wildlife sightings. Yesterday a huge bobcat slowly crossed the road in front of our car. It was the biggest one either Gene or I had ever seen, and its tail was long enough that for a moment I was confused and wanted to call out, "Mountain lion!" However, much as I want to see one of the fabled big cats (some deny there are any in this area, others swear to having seen one), it was clear on more careful examination that this was just a wonderfully robust bobcat. When we stopped the car, he scampered up the bank and sat gazing at us through the dried brush.

I saw a black squirrel on Edkin Hill Road. A lovely red fox with an unbelievably fat and bushy tail darted across the bridge that divides the Outlet Pond from the lake. And one morning last week, several hours before daybreak, I was awakened by the howling of coyotes. What an eerie, lonely sound. This was a first for me, although Craig and Dee, with a cabin more deeply in the woods, have heard them often. One ran across the road in front of Craig's truck, but I'm not sure I've ever seen one. However, there was that time at the airport, just at dusk, when something large and doglike trotted through the far end of the field, but I was not close enough to say for sure that it was a coyote. Gene and I love living close to all that's wild. We humans have such need of things, but these creatures of the forest sketch beauty in a life drawn from the basics.

The whole town has kept track of the twin albino fawns that appeared this spring in the fields behind Pete Rider's. Amazing photographs of them in all stages of growth are tacked to bulletin boards in JR'S convenience store and the local real estate office. In these snapshots, we see them as little things standing at their mother's side, later as strapping young bucks with their antlers all in velvet. Although most of the local folk are hunters, no one wants to see them fall to deer season. There is something mythic about these two, and if they get shot, it will be by outsiders.

I hate hunting season. The woods around us ring with the sound of gun-shots. But it is part of the price I pay for all this beauty. Up here, the year is not measured off spring, summer, fall, and winter. Instead folks speak of spring turkey season, small-game season, antlered and antlerless deer season, fall turkey and bear seasons, to name but a few of the more obvious ones. I'm afraid of guns. At the sound of the first shot, Carol, Chuckles, and I don flo-rescent orange vests for our morning runs. Craig and his coworkers are all of hunting stock. I am an embarrassment to this son of mine when hunting season comes. "Mom," he tells me in dismay, "you don't have to wear a vest. No one is going to shoot you on the road. The guys up here know how to hunt." I explain that it's not the local people that worry me but the flat-landers who have no hunting ethic. It falls on deaf ears. Carol and I are out on the road at just the hour these men report to work, and they all see us. Craig must take some teasing. "You're getting to be just like Bernadette," he tells me, referring to one older year-round summer person who wears her blaze orange vest when she walks the block and a half from her house to the post office. At least Carol and I run through forested areas where hunting does take place, but Craig won't yield the point. My vest is an insult to the skills of local hunters.

Anxious as I am to be done with my chemotherapy, I no longer cry when low white counts delay the recommended schedule. I hate cisplatin so much that I am always happy and grateful when the doctor sends me home untreated. A reprieve, a stay of execution! One more week of feeling mostly okay. I increasingly rely on my herbs and teas for peace of mind. I tell myself I'm treating the cancer even when the doctors can't. And, in fact, it seems to be true. I can no longer feel the mass in my lower right side. I decide that I have much to be thankful for in this month of thanksgiving.

Last year Gene and I hosted Thanksgiving for all the Carberry clan at our place in Osprey Lakes. It was great fun. Large though the house is, we still had to run two shifts, one for those who arrived the night before and one for those who stayed over the following evening. We filled all the bedrooms twice. We were twenty-five in all, if one counts Spike, the cat. Somehow, I miscalculated and laid one extra place. Spike gladly filled in, positioning himself at the head of the table, one front leg extended on the left-hand side of the plate, another on the right. Gene and I have always had what we refer to as the "two-foot rule" when it comes to cats joining us at the dinner table. They are allowed to sit in a chair, sit in front of a plate, and they may put their two front feet on the table, but nothing more. The rule has been quickly grasped by all of them. At the first sign of a back paw inching up there, they are immediately excused from the table. Spike, however, has taken advantage of his venerable age to push the rule to the limits. He often stretches his entire body across the table with only his back paws dangling off the edge. He is very fresh and, if not provided with a plate of his own, will reach one front paw out to snatch something from his nearest neighbor.

This year, knowing that chemotherapy might lay me low in the days before the holiday, I was afraid to commit to Thanksgiving. As it turns out, I get no treatment in November other than routine blood tests and Neupogen shots and am feeling as well as I have felt in months on Thanksgiving Day. But it has already been decided that we will gather at my sister Sandy's house. Craig and Dee, Erin and Kyle, and Ingrid pile into the car with Gene and me. There will be over thirty Carberrys there. I adore every one. Eccentric to a person, we overlook all flaws and peculiarities and simply rejoice in our love for each other. This clan was a feuding clan in the past. As recently as two generations ago, there were insanely magnificent quarrels, but those of us who are left, perhaps because we witnessed the pain of all that fury, are one tightly knit bunch. There is no trace of spite or envy. The success of one enhances us all.

Sandy, who lives in a magnificent stone colonial farmhouse, is a widow whose veterinarian husband died of cancer four or five years ago. It is the first time I have been to Sandy's house since I was diagnosed with cancer, and I am embarrassed by my disease, feel it is somehow impolite of me to walk around as a reminder of all that she went through. Of course, no one else shows any signs of sharing my discomfort, and the day is one glorious celebration of all that is good in our lives. Sitting with my family at a long table in a house surrounded by farmland, barns, and Sandy's horses, sheep, and cows, there is very much an over-the-river-and-through-the-woods feel to the entire day. Sometimes I watch my life as though it were a play and wonder how it is I landed such a wonderful part.

Sandy has two beagles who have spent the day being so enthusiastic about what is in the oven that somewhere in the midst of the preparations, she removes them to an outside kennel. We are all inspired to recall past Thanksgivings with dogs. I think more canines get in trouble on this holiday than on any other day of the year. When we were girls, we had cocker spaniels. Our mother had much stricter rules about animals and food than I have ever been able to enforce. Dusky, our old cocker, was really good about obeying them. She had just finished raising a litter of pups on the Thanksgiving in question, so perhaps she can be forgiven for the transgressions of that year. Mother was in a frenzy of last-minute gravy-stirring, potato-mashing, and table-setting. She stepped away from her cooking to attend to something in the dining room, and we all heard a tremendous thud at her vacated spot in the kitchen. Dashing in there, we saw a completely unabashed Dusky dragging the roasted turkey by one leg across the kitchen floor. Mother, who had always been offended by people who allowed dogs to eat from human plates, amazed me by wrenching the turkey away from Dusky and hoisting it into the kitchen sink where she ran it under hot water. With all of us hungrily waiting, I guess she had no choice but to slice and serve all parts except the leg by which Dusky had done the dragging.

We were finally ready to sit down when Mother remembered the wine she had cooling in the unheated, enclosed porch just off the kitchen. She sent me to retrieve a bottle. Now there was more than wine on that porch. There were also four five-month-old cocker spaniel puppies, the remains of a litter that had not sold as well as Mother had hoped. I really did try to keep them in, but something in the smell of roasting turkey drives all dogs wild. Little Silver, true to the quicksilver aspects of her name, squeezed between my legs. She came charging through the kitchen and zoomed around the corner into the dining room as if she had been rehearsing the move for every day of a much longer life than the one she possessed. Somewhere in the doorway that divided the two rooms, she took flight and vaulted with Olympian grace in a long arching leap that landed her squarely in the dish of mashed potatoes. I think she was aiming for the turkey, but she fell a little short. I have no memory of what followed, but I think it safe to guess we did without potatoes that year.

Craig and Dee's old Newfoundland, Vern, never left the yard. He required no watching at all. One Thanksgiving, Dee got a call from Ben Roberts, who owns one of the condominiums on the hill 150 yards above Dee's house. Now Ben has a reputation for being somewhat fond of his after-dinner brandy, and Dee was quite certain he had taken advantage of the holiday and indulged in a few extra rounds, for he was insisting that Vern had stolen the rather considerable remains of his Thanksgiving turkey. It seems he had put it on the front porch to cool, not exactly a clever move in this land of marauding skunks, opossums, raccoons, and bears. Ben, no small man himself, described wrestling with a huge black creature over ownership of the bird. Dee wondered if it might not have been a bear that had finally wandered off in triumphant possession of all but the left leg. "It couldn't have been Vern," she protested. "He's right out here in the yard." As she was talking on the phone, she walked over to the window to test the proof of her assertion. And, indeed, she was right. Vern *was* lying out there in their yard—happily gnawing on a large, golden brown turkey.

Winter is settling in. The ground is frozen. We've had our first snowfalls, the sky holds steady with the leaden gray I find so comforting. Gene and Craig have hung the heavy, old wooden storm windows. The woodstove is cleaned and ready for nonstop service right into April. We always stock up on a season's supply of firewood in November. Willis, who prides himself on delivering beautifully split and stacked, clean, dry hardwood, doesn't like to make the trip up the mountain in winter. He correctly observes, "The trouble with snow in Osprey Lakes is that when it snows in Osprey Lakes, it hain't got the sense to melt." We feel lucky to be on the list of those for whom he will provide. Willis cares about his product and won't bring wood to anyone who won't store it in a dry place out of the weather. We are fortunate to have large porches that meet the specifications for shelter.

Now on this particular day, I hear Willis's truck pull up in front of the house at 6:30 A.M. Surprised that he isn't unloading, I turn on the porch light and go out to see if there is some problem. Indeed, there is. To back his truck directly up to our front porch, he must drive across four feet of the next-door neighbor's yard. Anthea is a snowbird who heads for Florida at the first sign of frost. One of Anthea's blue spruce trees has grown so large over the summer that Willis is afraid one especially long branch will scratch the side of his truck. "Do you think I could just saw this one branch off?" Willis asks, already reaching into the back for the saw he keeps handy for emergencies such as this.

"Oh, boy, Willis," I say. "I don't know. That's not my tree. I don't think we ought to do that."

"Well, that branch could pretty much ruin a feller's truck."

I look at it more closely, argue for a slightly different angle of approach. Willis stands firm. The branch has to go. Finally I relent, but not really much. Holding up the bough in question, I allow that it is a little longer than its companions. "Perhaps we could just prune it a bit." I indicate the place where we could unobtrusively snip it back the necessary three inches. He raises the saw. "Oh, no, Willis," I tell him. "I'll do it. Let me go down in the basement and get my pruning shears." I really do hurry as fast as I can, but by the time I return, Willis has sawed off the branch in question right back to the trunk. Not only that, but he has also taken every other branch on that side of the tree from the five-foot-mark right down to the ground. I am aghast, absolutely stunned. From where I stand, the formerly stately blue spruce looks like a palm tree. I love Willis and have never criticized him, but this time I cry out in pain, "Oh, Willis, no!"

He looks at me just ever so slightly chagrined. "Well, once I took that one branch off, them there others just didn't look right."

I understand the seriousness of the crime Willis and I have committed. My decision not to call Anthea and inform her of the tragedy is not based solely on cowardice. I see no point in spoiling her Christmas, her lovely winter season in Florida. There is so much else that is going to wait until spring. The tree will wait as well. I think Anthea and I will eventually recover, although I am afraid that an entire summer may pass before she will be able to look at me without being reminded of the lopsided state of her tree.

Granddaddy Carberry, my mother's father, wouldn't own a dog that didn't bite. He took enormous pride in close relationships with animals that struck terror in the hearts of others. Only Granddaddy Carberry could get past Roughneck the rooster to gather the eggs. When Granddaddy was not around, my mother would engage Roughneck in battle with a long-handled mop while my sisters and I darted by them to raid the nest boxes. Granddaddy's dogs bit; his cats scratched; his horses kicked; and Reggie, the Scotch Highland ram with the curling rack of horns, could send anyone of any size sailing twenty feet through the air.

As a child I was as stubbornly angry as any of Granddaddy's animals. Ingrid loves to go through the family albums and point out photos of me scowling. "Oh, Mommy," she says with admiration, "you were tough."

"I was an awful child," I admit. "I always complained that no one loved me, but how could they, really? Look at that unhappy face. Only Granddaddy Carberry made me feel truly adored no matter what I did."

"What do you mean, no matter what you did?" Ingrid laughs. "He loved you because of what you did. You were just one more critter in his mean barnyard."

Chapter 8

December

I am counting now on every ounce of meanness I can muster. I am determined to butt and kick and bite and scratch my way to the finish here. They nail me again in early December. I am so rocked by the treatment that I propose new terms to Dr. Silverman, and he readily agrees. In the week following a chemotherapy session, I will return to the hospital every other day for IV infusions of fluids and Zofran, a powerful antinausea drug that is, at this point, available only intravenously. Cisplatin is hard on the kidneys. The medical profession gets around this problem by accompanying cisplatin treatments with eight hours of IV fluids. They always send me home with the admonition to drink lots of liquids, but I am unable to keep even sips of water down once the effect of the Zofran wears off. This new schedule will deal with both the fluids issue and the nausea. Nothing seems to deal with the two weeks of deep bodily unease, a sense that all is awry with me, out of sync, out of kilter, every internal rhythm missing a beat, faltering, misfiring.

Add the fatigue inspired by low white counts to the equation, and I am having trouble envisioning how I will manage the Christmas holidays. I did take advantage of a treatment-free November to begin preparations. Every year, I promise our grown children that I will keep it simple. My intentions are always honest, but every year I get carried away by the excess that defines

Christmas in our house. I who am such a penny-pincher the rest of the year abandon all restraint in December.

Fearful of infection, I've been doing all my shopping through mail-order catalogs. One day Chuckles and I are walking the snowy path around the lake when we unexpectedly encounter a friend who is himself a cancer survivor. He asks how I'm doing, and I reply, "Okay, you know, I have to be careful to stay out of crowds and stuff." He gestures at the frozen sweep of isolation before us and says, "Tough to do in Osprey Lakes, isn't it?"

I do love winter. Before the lake freezes, ice forms gleaming orbs that cling to the hemlock branches that hang low over the surface and are splashed by its waters. Every morning, from the upstairs bathroom window I check the progress of the skim of ice that makes its way under the footbridge and out across the lake. The cold can be brutal in December, but as long as there is a strong wind, the lake keeps some open water. Our house is positioned at the southern end of the lake. When the wind whips in from the north, it drives a fine powder of snow dust in around the windows on the closed-for-the-season sunporch. The whole house shakes and moans. I get up early every morning to fire the woodstove. My goal is not to have to start a fire from scratch until I close the system down in spring.

Because I live here alone except for weekends, I am the mechanic of the house. I understand its idiosyncrasies in a way that Gene does not. Until we bought Fitch Cottage, it had never been occupied in the winter months. These old houses were all summer cottages, designed for July and August living. As a result, they are far better at staying cool than they are at staying warm. The first winter we were here, we had one of the coldest Decembers on record, and everything froze. Every year since then, we've done a bit of insulating, but that first December, I had to get up several times each night to run water through all the spigots if I wanted to avoid frozen pipes in the morning. And even then, I called the Housts, our local plumbing dynasty, several times a week for help.

The Housts are a family worth knowing. They are not a clan given to display, and strangers make the mistake of underestimating the formidable IQs that are this family's genetic marker. Larry likes his beer, therefore his skills are more reliable in the morning than in the afternoon. One of the boys worked for NASA for a while, but missed the mountain and came home to the family business. Ronnie keeps a low profile and may be best known for pants that appear always in danger of falling off. The father, Gus, delights me by riding the only one-speed bike in town that is as least as old and beat-up as my own. When not on the bike, his two other transportation alternatives are a late-model Cadillac and an elaborate motor home.

Gus has mostly ceded the business to his sons, but that first year, he was still on call. The Housts have keys to almost every house in town. Minutes within my phoning, I often heard them moving through the basement or the upstairs bathrooms. The problem would be fixed and they'd be gone without my ever having seen them. I called the Housts so often in the first weeks of that cold December that I established a pattern that caused concern when it was broken. I bumped into Gus in the post office, and he looked rather worried when he asked if I was okay. I assured him that I was, and he explained, "Well, you haven't called us in two weeks, and we were afraid that something had happened to you." Something had: I'd learned how to thaw my own pipes.

Was it possible to winterize this house? That first December, we mostly winterized ourselves, pulling on long underwear and enough layers of turtlenecks and woolen sweaters to insure comfort in any outside venture. Except, of course, that we weren't dressing for the out-of-doors but for our living room! One local contractor bet me a steak dinner that I wouldn't last through a single winter. I laughed. "I can't take your money that easily. You obviously don't know me or you'd understand that stubbornness will carry me through the first winter. You can take me out to dinner when I've made it through two."

A year ago, our old cat, Spike, fell prey to a December blizzard. It was a tragedy for all of us that we tried to soften by focusing on what a lovely Thanksgiving he'd had. Gene and I were both glad we hadn't forced him from his place at the head of the table. The snow was just starting, and I stood at the door bidding an extended farewell to Dee (we always think of one more story we have to share). Spike must have slipped out unnoticed. Just before we went to bed, Gene asked, "Where's Spike?" We hunted through the house for half an hour before the awful truth dawned. We called and searched and tried to track his footprints, but the wind blew our voices back in our faces as surely as the snow covered any trace of his passage. I grabbed a flashlight, put on snowshoes, and took Chuckles through the woods in search. Gene walked the roads, looking under every bush. When all that failed, he climbed in the car and inched his way around the lake, calling, "Kitty, kitty," out the opened window. Sometime after midnight, we gave up and went to bed heartsick.

Early the next morning, we resumed the search, but Spike had vanished so without a trace that I feared he was either frozen in some snowbank or had been carried off in the talons of a great horned owl. We tried to console ourselves. He was fourteen. He'd had a perfect life, filled with joy and freedom, far better to die of adventure than of old age.

Gene gave up hope before I did. Ten days after Spike's disappearance, I still spent most of every dog walk calling, "Here, Spikey, Spike, Spike. Here kitty, kitty." Gene pleaded with me to stop. "This is getting to be like *Come Back, Little Sheba*. Please just let me bury this cat, mourn, and recover." But, burdened with the guilt of the long good-bye, I could not. It rained. It froze. A heavy crust formed on the snow. We had notices posted in the papers and all over town. Eventually I began to give up hope. Spike was such a smart cat. Even though all his familiar landmarks were covered by four feet of snow that might not melt until spring, I couldn't understand why, if he was alive, he hadn't found his way back to us.

And then one night we had a light dusting of snow, barely enough to sweep across the frozen crust and gather around windbreaks such as houses. Just as I was finishing writing one afternoon, I got a call from Fred, who lives over near the beach. He had seen cat tracks around his house when he'd gotten up that morning. He cautioned me against false hope. "There is a feral cat that raised kittens in the woods behind my house last summer. It's probably one of them."

Gene had called from Philly to ask me to wait to walk the dog until he got there. He pulled in just as I was gathering Chuckles and snowshoes together to go check out this one last hope. Neither one of us wanted to let ourselves believe, and yet when we saw the prints, my heart beat faster. What cat but Spike sported such a big, round foot? Fred, an accomplished naturalist, had already eliminated the possibility that it might be a bobcat. I put my finger in the print and gave Chuckles the old tracking command, "Find it. Find it." The minute he first snorted his nose into the snow, his whole posture changed, and he took off in an excited circle that looped him through the woods and back to Fred's house, then off down the ice-packed lane. I scrambled to get my snowshoes on in time to follow him. I clomped after him on the top crust of frozen fields, waving my arms and crying out, "Find it. Find it."

We charged along parallel to the road where Gene walked, muttering, as he later admitted, to himself, "Crazy broad! She won't give up until we've gone to every house in Osprey Lakes."

Chuckles did follow the trail up onto the front porch of every boarded-up and shuttered summer house. Spike has a reputation for making himself comfortable around town. He knows how to open the screen doors of most of these old homes, and he lets himself in and takes over pretty much when and where he pleases. One woman awoke from a nap to find him asleep on the pillow beside her head. Another man, who was having his morning coffee, saw Spike arrogantly stroll through their kitchen on what was not our pet's first visit to the home and complained to his wife, "That damned cat thinks he owns this house." I'm afraid that the gentleman was correct in his assessment. Spike did think he owned a large number of the homes in town. So, I was heartened by the route this trail was taking and called out through happy tears to Gene, "I know this is Spike. I know it is. What other cat would try to open every door?" I consider all animals capable of the miraculous. Gene, protecting himself against the pain of disappointment, was more willing to believe that his wife had finally lost her mind.

Meanwhile, Chuckles and I forged ahead. We scrambled across frozen streams, and through the woods and fields. Just often enough to reinforce my confidence in the talent lodged in this dog's nose, we came to a spot where the blown dust of snow had gathered in one place and held the clear print of a cat's paw. Only when we came to plowed roads or driveways did Chuckles lose the trail. Then he would cast up and down along the side of the road until he found it again. Up over the snowbank he would go, with me calling encouragement to both dog and man. "Find it. Find it. He's on the trail again, Gene! He's on the trail!"

Finally, about a mile from our starting place, Chuckles ran in under a porch and moved two garbage cans aside with his body. (For me, this is the most amazing part of the story. Chuckles is so prissy that he refuses to move through any doorway unless the door is opened wide enough that it doesn't touch him.) But he just pushed those two old galvanized tins over, and out stepped Spike! Chuckles had led me directly to him! I cried out to Gene, "We found him! We found him!" but I was sobbing so hard that Gene was certain Spike was dead and it was the remains we had found. And, in truth, what remained of Spike was not much. Our normally plump cat was bone thin, his skin sort of dry and wrinkled, hanging around the splendid creature that he used to be but was no more. Two weeks in the bitter, frozen landscape. How had he done it?

Chuckles was so excited that he leaped higher than my head, reaching out with his long tongue to kiss Spike, whom I held in my arms, on both the way up and the way down. What a triumphant procession we made walking down the road toward home! Chuckles pranced in front, head held high, chest thrown out, tail a mighty waving standard. He knew he was a hero. There was pride telegraphed in every step. It was his moment of glory. For once he had driven his much immortalized predecessor, Scoobie, into the background. The moment belonged to Chuckles, and he clearly knew it. Gene and I took turns carrying Spike, and every now and then Chuckles would come back to nuzzle and check Spike over. This old cat had raised Chuckles from a pup. Spike has always had a nursemaid quality to him. He is our caretaker, but now it was his turn for royal treatment.

Once home, we settled him on fluffed pillows, offered water and tidbits of food. He drank but seemed to know not to eat too much. For the first twenty-four hours he was home, he did not sleep but sat with the wide-eyed, shocked expression of someone who had been slapped with terror. And then, once that first day and night were over, he relaxed into the security of home, sleeping purring, with his soft, exposed belly turned up to all the love we lavished on him. Within a week, the only sign of his trauma was a leaner, more svelte profile. All things are possible. My animals have taught me that.

This December is a hard one for reasons that have nothing to do with weather. Too many packages to wrap, too many phone calls, too many parties, too many cards, too much of everything in a season that always over-whelms me but this year appears to have my complete destruction in mind. Why can't I just say no? I don't understand it myself. This year I have my illness as a ready-made alibi, but I am unable to use it. I seem determined to present myself as being in far better health than I am, to prove that cancer has not stopped me, will not stop me.

Gene and I have a friend. No, he is more than a friend. Even though there is no genetic or legal basis, Tyrone is family. He will be fifteen on Christmas Day. I first met Ty when he was six years old and the playmate of a little boy who lived on our street in Philadelphia. Moving away from Tyrone was one of the hardest parts about leaving the city and coming to Osprey Lakes. Now I fear that the chaos of this holiday season will jeopardize the only present he has asked for this year (but not the only one he will get). In response to my plea for gift ideas, he wrote me a touching letter of several pages, insisting on every one that my only gift be a complete recovery. "All I want is that you, Heather Trexler Remoff, get better. You have to beat that old cancer. You have to keep that stubborn way about you to fight it off. That is a great quality. That's all I want for Christmas and my birthday. That is all!" I love him so much. I know that his request is one that the rest of my family shares. Why do I put it all at risk by letting myself be consumed by the season?

My walks with Chuckles are my only slice of serenity. But I can't take the cold the way I used to, and by the time I get myself sufficiently bundled, walking itself is difficult. The lake froze early in the month. This is always a holy moment for me. Ice had steadily been creeping in from the edges for weeks. It was cold enough, but the world remained too filled with move-ment. And then one late afternoon, the wind just stopped. The silence was breathtaking, and I knew that by morning the lake would be transformed. Icy winter—with its spare, crystalline beauty defined by the very lack of a liv-ing, breathing pulse—now holds dominion here.

I heard that Peter, who owns one of the old inns in town, swam in the days just before the lake froze. Now only February eludes him. Peter has been swimming in this lake in every month but that one. There was a year when two weeks of unseasonable warmth in January forced a partial thaw, and Peter took quick advantage of the freak weather to extend his record. Gene and I are impressed. Peter and his wife bought the inn not long after we moved to town. We are glad that eccentricity is not confined to those with roots going back some generations. Much as I love the winter, I secretly hope for a temporary February thaw, so that Peter will have done it all. He refuses to cut a hole in the ice, but chooses, instead, to take advantage of suddenly presented opportunities. Last February, Chuckles fell through the ice where the sun-warmed supports holding the footbridge had created a weak spot. Gene's immediate response to the temporary calamity faced by his dog was "Quick, go get Peter!" But the hole in the ice made access to a spot that was not deep enough to offer any danger to Chuckles or any opportunity to really swim, and so February remains elusive.

Fitch Cottage is so beautiful, so made for Christmas, that it is hard to imagine that, until we moved here, it had stood for over one hundred years cold and abandoned during the holiday season. Gene and I ring the outside porches with garlands of white pine. We loop boxwood and lemons along the banisters of the stately staircase and over the arcades that separate living, dining, entry, and game room areas. The mantelpiece is covered with evergreens brought in from the yard and forest. I make enormous wreaths to hang on the front door and on the upstairs, outside wall facing the street. There are candles everywhere.

We cut our tree from a plantation down in Glen Mawr or Mawr Glen. No one seems quite sure of the name of the town. When you enter from the east, the highway marker claims one name, a different one from that declared when you enter from the west. I let the local bar resolve the issue. The neon sign of the Glen Mawr Hotel tells me all I need to know. The trees are all Fraser fir, a lovely deep green with needles short and dense and soft. Every year we decorate our tree with gingerbread men, honeycakes, popcorn and cranberry chains, and real candles instead of strings of lights. Or I should say Ingrid and I put candles on the tree. Gene is so terrified of the whole enterprise that his self-assigned role is to stand by with a full bucket of water whenever Ing and I reach for the matches. When he's around, the candles stay lit only long enough for us to take some hurried photographs. I'm convinced there is far less danger from candles than from electric lights. First of all, a tree this fresh and green would be hard to set on fire even if that were one's intent. But beyond that, people are careless with electricity, leaving the tree illuminated when they go out or off to bed. We never leave the room when our tree is alive and flickering with the soft glow of all those tiny flames.

We like to have our big meal on Christmas Eve. That way the day itself can be devoted to slowly and lovingly opening gifts and visiting with each other. We take frequent breaks to graze among the leftovers from the previous night's feast. The "kids," as our adult children have resigned themselves to being called, always contribute to the Christmas Eve dinner, but this year I have been forbidden to assist in the preparations in any way. They insist on doing everything. I am assigned duty resting on the couch.

It is just starting to snow when Ingrid and John arrive. The ground is already covered with a foot or more. "Ah, Christmas in Bavaria," Ingrid calls to me as she gets out of the car. She and John are both loaded down with grocery bags and gaily wrapped packages. Dana and Derek, each with a sleeping baby in their arms, show up not long afterward. Leighanne pops awake as soon as the cold hits her, but we manage to get Cody into one of the upstairs bedrooms to finish his nap. Craig and Dee and Erin and Kyle have been darting in and out all week. The air is charged with secrets, the wait for the big day interminable for these little ones. Everyone is determined to help, and I feel like a queen ruling from my pallet and basking in the glow from the fireplace while the kitchen fills up with wonderful aromas.

Suddenly we notice that Leighanne is missing. A hurried search locates her in the closed-off bedroom that I have used as a hiding place. I have been diligent in a way not usual for me. Knowing my limitations, I had dutifully wrapped each mail-ordered gift as soon as it arrived. Leighanne has found them all and sits joyously engaged in a sea of torn paper and ribbons. The damage looks worse initially than it actually is. Her parents grab her and, along with everyone else, hurry back downstairs to the stirring and cooking. I am left to try to match name tags to presents. I know this is a funny story, a tale that will be told with laughter time and time again, the stuff of family legend. But I am weeping as I rewrap and patch the packages together. And I hate my cancer then as I have never hated it before. Has it robbed me of my soul, my humor, all grandmotherly affection?

The meal itself is a triumph, everything so gleaming and lovely that it drives the last trace of self-pity from me. My great-aunt Kate's silver compote is filled with polished nuts and small fruits that would be exotic in any season but seem near miraculous in this land of snow. Mother's white linen tablecloth highlights the cobalt blue and gold of the china plates that had been the pride and joy of the old Lakeside Hotel. The hotel was torn down in the sixties, but its spirit fills the room tonight. We hold my grandmother's crystal goblets aloft, toasting each other, the future, and all that has gone before us. Ingrid starts the feast with my favorite herbed oysters baked on the half shell. The rest of the meal is a happy blur: Dana's salad, Derek's green beans with onions and red peppers, Craig's done-to-perfection roast, Dee's twice-baked potatoes piled high and crusted with cheese and paprika, homemade bread, and for dessert our traditional finish, a yule log so exquisitely decorated with tiny meringue mushrooms, chocolate acorns, berries, and live greens that it seems the work of fairies, surely not something we can actually eat.

I finish the year happy but exhausted. How can even love joyously and freely given drain me so?

My father was a great believer in discipline as long as it was practiced by other people. When I was twelve, he launched a campaign to remake my mother. For months on end we heard lectures on the importance of high fiber, deep breathing, vigorous walking, sleeping with the windows open. The fact that my father failed to practice what he preached did not in any way dampen the strength of his convictions and was probably responsible for the increasingly high volume with which he made his pitch. Mother's idea of recreation was a cigarette and a book. Her unresponsiveness to his badgering culminated in the episode that finally silenced him. She clipped a terse poem from McCall's magazine and taped it to the mirror above his dresser.

> *You go exercise*
> *You go diet*
> *You go breathe deep*
> *I just want quiet.*

Chapter 9

January

January is the quiet month, possessed of an ice-blue purity. This clean asceticism is a welcome relief after the scarlet excess of December. December has always been too much for me, but this year I was overly concerned with demonstrating to the world that I was okay. As a result, I feel dangerously exhausted.

I can't remember the name of the author who described himself as a gregarious recluse, but I will ever be grateful to him. The phrase lodged immediately in my psyche. It was as if, after having suffered elusive physical complaints for years, I finally found a doctor able to put a name to the syndrome. It didn't matter that no cure was offered. There was comfort in the sudden absence of ambiguity. A gregarious recluse. With those words, I knew myself and understood why the gaiety of December was so draining to my spirit. Some people love the holidays and are nourished by them. I too love the gathering in of family, the search for just the perfect gift to delight a cherished person, the wrapping of presents, the aroma of cinnamon, the warmth of the oven with its offerings of food. But I am not nourished by December. I am emptied out, hollowed, held together by a veneer so thin, so brittle, that the movement even of dance could shatter me.

Luckily, January comes just in time to offset December's intoxicating immersion in the social. Like a long period of fasting following a diet of chocolate, cheese, and gravy, January purifies. It would, of course, be healthier to strike a daily balance between the gregarious and reclusive aspects of myself, but I have never been able to negotiate with December. I simply wait for January to heal me.

Perhaps the only difficult aspect of the month is being pulled from sleep by the alarm in a room so dark that it could as easily be 2 as 5:30 A.M. This is one of civilization's most barbaric moments. I can't believe it's healthy. But we let our schedules rule our lives, and mine is run by the clock almost as completely as that of someone who reports to an office. The alarm is always set to allow for precious minutes in the charmed space between sleep and wakefulness. Ideas run in and out of my head, some utterly wacky with the strange distortion of logic and sequence so common to dreams. Others stay with me and later get reworked into theories that delight me with their streamlined clarity. I take great pleasure from these early-morning "insights" even though I am aware that what appears clear to me is often viewed by others as bizarre.

The sound of the alarm is so harsh. It dislodges any sleep-won serenity. And this is true despite the fact that I have selected a model with a relatively soft tone. People have suggested clock radios to me, but I trust no station's choice of music to be appropriate for waking, and even the possibility of a commercial jarring me out of sleep is enough to discourage me from pursuing that option. Gene is my second husband. When we were first married, he liked to wake to a twenty-four-hour news station. He abandoned it after a few episodes of my unconsciously mixing "creative insights" with actual news stories. The children were in high school. Gene was an executive in a busy corporate headquarters. I would send them out the door in the morning with news on the latest breaking stories. Bombings, assassinations of top politicians, the discovery of vast reserves of oil in a neighboring town. I was convincing because of the totality of my own belief. I had "heard" it on the news just that morning. It was only after they had repeated my dramatic updates to people who had heard the real news or who raced to the TV to gather more information that my total lack of early-morning credibility was exposed. We weren't married very many months before Gene traded the clock radio for a conventional alarm.

I wish someone would design a humane alarm, one that is sensitive to our deepest biological rhythms. I'm convinced that we aren't meant to wake up until the sun rises. Winter is supposed to be a time for long hours of sleep, shortened work hours. Surely there would be less depression if we adjusted our cycles of sleep and wakefulness to accommodate the hours of naturally available light. Wouldn't those afflicted with seasonal affective disorder, a type of depression treated by exposure to lamps that mimic the wavelengths of naturally occurring light, benefit just as much from nights that simply allowed more sleep? But we are no longer hunters and gatherers or Stone Age farmers, and the corporate world has its own ideas about what constitutes a good night's sleep. I think the solution is in an alarm that mimics dawn in the same way that those lamps mimic natural light.

In the spring, the barest murmurings of birdsong precede the first light. My clock would start with sweet sound so low as to be only subliminally audible. A chirp or two and then silence, a hint of ruffling feathers shifting on a branch. More silence. And then a fine ribbon of light, something midnight soft, a mere shading away from black. And gradually, gradually the song would increase in volume and complexity. As it did, the lamp would cast tones of peach and gold until finally the room would fill with bright light and a chorus of birdsong. That is how I would prefer to wake up, but January does not accommodate me.

I like my bedroom very cold. Even now, when chemotherapy has sucked all warmth from my marrow, I can't give up the old habits. It is not cold enough unless a glass of water left on the windowsill has a thin skim of ice on it by morning. I love to feel the condensed substance of my breath in the dark above my face, but my body must be toasty. I take strange delight in putting a sleep-warmed hand up to touch a frosty cheek and nose. The secret to this perfect mix of fire and ice is goose down. My great-grandmother's four-poster bed is fat as a marshmallow. Every morning I fluff the feather bed into a great airy mound, all the while anticipating sinking into its welcoming loft come nightfall. On top of this puff of feathers goes a thick goose-down quilt. Before going to bed, I warm two old firebricks on the woodstove for an hour or two. Shortly before retiring, I tuck these hot bricks between the feather bed and the quilt. When I finally climb in, a heavenly sea of warmth is waiting for me, an oasis of pure comfort in the center of that frigid room.

One reason that I get up so early is that Carol and I stick to our 7 A.M. running schedule regardless of the weather. I like to have all my morning tasks behind me before leaving the house. That way, I return to a clean slate with less to distract me on my way from the shower to the typewriter.

Once Chuckles and I step out the door, I understand why I continue to set the alarm for five-thirty. The first breath of air is immediately cold. All sensation is distilled into the simple fact of existence. Even Chuckles leaps with a joy more pronounced than that of any other season. I glory in the thrill of movement in an otherwise still world. Our house faces east. Venus remains low on the horizon and in early January hangs just under a sliver of moon. The stark outlines of trees are edged with the first pale hints of morning light. Venus was there in December, but I paid it no heed. Now I scan the sky eagerly and am calm at the core the instant its steady light and I connect. "We may take something like a star," I tell myself in Robert Frost's words, "to stay our minds on and be staid."

The cold makes me feel light, fit, and fast, but it is all a lie, an illusion that Carol helps reinforce. Almost nine months into my chemotherapy treatments, I know that I used to walk faster than I am now running. Carol, always lean and quick, could run rings around me even in my best days, but now she matches her pace to mine with never a word. Sometimes I glance at her from the corner of my eye, study her form. How does she do it, manage to look as if we are running when it probably takes us fifteen minutes to cover a mile? I should tell her how much I love her but instead I bitch about my bone marrow. "These white counts are killing me. At the rate I'm going, they'll never give me my last treatment." It's not that I really want the treatment, but I desperately need all of this to be over. "If I can just get the count up to three, I think they'll go ahead."

"Ah, why don't you wait a week or two. The ice is almost ready now." Carol knows how to hook me. January is the month for serious ice-watching. As soon as the ice is twelve or more inches thick, the town will spend the weekend building Osprey Lakes' famous ice toboggan slide. It's such a unique event that this tiny borough was once featured on *Good Morning America*. Carol knows that I will be in no condition to harvest ice if I indulge in cisplatin cocktails in the few weeks preceding slide construction.

I'm eager for all the details. Carol, who has lived in Osprey Lakes for twenty-seven years, has a direct line to slide information. "Smitty measured it last night. If it stays cold, they hope to build it next weekend." The vagaries of weather add to the charm of slide construction. One year a heavy blanket of snow insulated the ice and kept it from reaching the necessary thickness.

Our run is almost over. I do only one lap around the lake, have promised my doctors to keep my daily jog in the neighborhood of two miles. In the beginning, I chaffed at this limitation, but now it is a promise that is ever easier to keep. I have a reputation for being a headstrong patient. They have no idea of how cowed I have become. I seem to spend my life doing what I'm told. Naps. Fluids. Neupogen shots. Blood tests. A fearful avoidance of crowds and their potential germs. What has happened to the world's healthiest woman? I pull my wool cap down around my ears, another concession I make to cancer. I've never worn a hat, but now the thin covering of hair that graces my head offers no protection. "What's the weather report?" I ask Carol before she moves off on her second lap. "Cold and colder," she calls back over her shoulder.

The thermometer proves her right. By afternoon, the red line of mercury drops quickly past ten degrees on its way to zero. Gene and I bundle ourselves to the point of mummies for our afternoon walk with Chuckles. We head out a little early, before the cold becomes any more bitter. My body has lost a lot of its heat-generating capacity. I even tie a wool scarf across my face, bank-robber fashion. Chuckles races madly about our feet. As soon as we hit the Laurel Path, he dives into a snowbank and sends two fat grouse thundering into the air. When it is this cold, grouse will burrow into the insulating protection of the snow. Following our field dog's rude intrusion, they land in low hemlock branches, sending down a fine white dusting. Chuckles explodes into action. Black dog, white snow, and holy winter shatter every hold my failing body has on me. Somewhere I leave that wretched, broken thing behind me, and the rest of the walk is pure joy.

When the temperature drops this quickly, the lake sings. I've only heard recordings of whale song, never the real thing, but it is the analogy I use when trying to explain to anyone the haunting beauty of this phenomenon. It's a deep sound that echoes with subtle variations in tone and pitch as it rolls under the ice and across the lake. Is there something lost and prehistoric trapped there? I once wrote to our weather channel asking for an explanation. I got one by return mail. Why can I not remember the science of the learned meteorologist's response? On a cold, clear night when the wind is

still, we can stand on our porch and hear that lonesome calling. It has a res-
onant, otherworldly quality, nothing that could possibly be explained by air
bubbles and quickly shifting shelves of ice.

At last, the notice goes up on the post office bulletin board. All systems are
go for slide-building. Smitty is the undisputed authority on the construction.
He is a tall man, broad-shouldered, taciturn. I confess to being a little bit
afraid of him. He is so no-nonsense, his authenticity intimidates me. This is
his world. I'm too newly here to lay claim to it. Just by opening my mouth,
I can reveal myself as a frivolous pretender, a "flatlander." I've never had a
real conversation with Smitty, but there must be someone who has. Because,
in January, most of the exchanges overheard in the post office start with the
phrase "Smitty says." He and the select few with real expertise in this eso-
teric art begin work the Friday before. That is when the ice field is plowed,
measured, scored, and cut to within an inch of the unfrozen depths. The
slide was first built in 1904. Knowledge of how to do so is handed down. It
is not unusual to work beside someone whose slide-building heritage goes
back three generations. The basic design and method of construction remain
essentially unchanged.

Whenever I ride the slide, I am certain I will be killed before the wooden
toboggan reaches the flat, smooth surface of the lake. It travels at speeds of
over forty miles an hour. There is no way to steer, and it keeps moving far
too fast for these old bones long after it hits the level surface of the frozen
lake. It terrifies me. Only the desire to participate in this community ritual
and the knowledge of the precision with which it is engineered enable me to
ease myself in behind my family members for a drop down a frozen channel on an out-of-control roller coaster plunging through a world of hard,
hard ice.

Our Place, one of the local restaurants, volunteers to feed all the workers breakfast at 6 A.M. Gene and I are dilettantes; we always take Chuckles
for his morning walk before proceeding to the ice field and have yet to appear at the breakfast. By the time we finally show up, it's 9 A.M., and the first
truckloads of ice have already been hauled to the base of the hill and reach
from the shore partway across the lake. We always work the field. There is

a fairly rigid, gender-based division of labor. The men do the marking and sawing. They direct the cut blocks onto the conveyor belt that carries them onto the trucks, and they always do the unloading. The blocks weigh at least 250 pounds and must be gripped and lifted with tongs in order to position them. I am told that this is the hardest job.

The power saw that makes the deep, rough cuts through the ice is one of the most frightening machines I have ever seen. Like all of the other equipment necessary to slide-building, it has been designed and made by the men of this community. Form follows function is sort of the basic law, but the resulting inventions bear so little relationship to the sleek, smooth lines of an Eames chair that the phrase takes on a whole new meaning. Rube Goldberg may be the inspiration here. It's hard not to wonder whose lawn mower is missing a motor, whose power saw has turned up without a blade?

The first year I helped with the slide, I inadvertently backed into the path of the monster saw. Now, I don't think they would deliberately halve someone who failed to yield, but the woman working next to me quickly pulled me to one side. A good thing, because as far as I could tell, there was no intention of slowing the saw. These folks are here to work, to build a toboggan slide, and novice volunteers quickly learn to master the task at hand or get out of the way. Aside from a few predictable laughs about slicing the bacon, this attempt at liposuction Sullivan County style passed without much notice or comment. There *is* a fierce beauty to the saw. The primitive rusty metal; the deafening, unmuffled roar; and the scowling focus of the man at the controls stand in sharp contrast to the dazzling loveliness of the shower of crystals it sprays behind. Hundreds of thousands of tiny shards of ice, each reflecting a pastel rainbow, spew out in its wake.

It remains bitter cold. Although it is not snowing, the wind is screaming in from the north and blowing so much loose snow with it that we are at times nearly blinded. Gene stands beside the conveyor, helping make sure the floating blocks hit it at the correct angle. Powered by an old tractor, the belt dips just below the surface of the water, gathering the floating blocks into place until they are released onto a sliding-board-like ramp that sends them skittering onto the waiting truck beds.

A long, narrow channel leads from the field to the shore and the waiting conveyor belt. The women of town line the channel and the open water of the area from which the ice has already been harvested. With long wooden harpoons in hand, we direct the free-floating ice from the field and down the sluice toward the trucks. This is a slow, cold process. "You know the reason they give us this job, don't you?" I ask the woman next to me. We are nearly unrecognizable to each other in our layers of hoods, scarves, coats, mittens, and boots. It is only when she answers that I am able to read her identity from her voice, muffled though it is by two wool scarves: "Body fat." We laugh and allow that the male contingent is sporting its share of beer bellies, but we don't see many of them reaching for harpoons. The water splashes up over our feet, and someone reminds us of the year one of the men slipped into the open water. I tell myself to be very careful. He was a longtime member of the community, and his misfortune is remembered mainly for its entertainment value. Were I to make such a splash, I fear the stories might have a different edge to them.

The first year I participated in a slide-building, I watched in fascination as the completion of the harvest was signaled by the positioning of blocks of ice at each of the four corners marking the open water of the now depleted field. "What do they do," I asked, "tie rope around the blocks so that no one falls in?"

"We don't need to do that," I was told. "Everybody knows we made the slide."

"But what about when it freezes?" I persisted. "You know, when the ice is still too thin to support someone's weight. What if someone was walking on the lake at night and fell through?"

There was a slight pause. "Only a flatlander would be dumb enough to do that."

I can feel myself getting way too cold, way too fast. Something is not right with me. I sense the concern of the women working on either side of me. Flatlander though I am, a large portion of the town has been solidly behind me in my battle against cancer. Casseroles and freshly baked loaves of bread are mysteriously waiting on the kitchen counter when I arrive home from a day at the hospital. Gene recently joked to a friend that if it was possible to time your illnesses in the right sequence, one would never have to cook in Osprey Lakes.

"Why don't you go over and stand by the fire for a while, drink some hot chocolate?"

"No, no. I'm okay, just a little cold. I need to move around a bit." I plunge my harpoon into a snowbank and try jumping up and down. It doesn't help much. I watch the men with envy. They are busy with their saws, their arms and bodies moving vigorously with each cut. Once all the long sides are cut through to the water, other men move behind them with custom-welded devices that bear a rough resemblance to crowbars and break that row free. I want one of those jobs, am convinced that all the activity would warm my bones. I don't think I'd have the strength and balance for the crowbar part of it. It seems a pretty sure way to sink to the bottom. But the sawing might be a different story. I wait till Bert Fiester pauses at the end of a row.

"Bert, can I try it for a minute or two? I just need to get warmed up." I have selected my quarry with care. Bert and his wife, Vera, have lived in town for years. They used to run the Sweet Shop. But that was before my time and before the time of many who are here today working on the slide. Not only is Bert well respected by everyone in town, but he is also a kind, gentle man, known for his helpfulness. He looks at me quizzically, but gives me a little grin and hands over the saw. To my surprise, the first pass of the saw is unbelievably easy. I'd forgotten that there was only an inch of ice to move through. So this is the secret the men have been keeping from the women! Cutting the ice is a snap, requiring no strength at all. Even I am able to do it with a fair degree of efficiency. However, once I get warmed up, I become uncomfortable with my break with tradition and thank Bert and reluctantly hand the saw back to him.

Someone has taken over my position with the harpoon. What am I doing here? I'm simply going through the motions. The truth is that the slide will get built without me. I wander back to my house and toss a few logs on the fire. With a deep sense of defeat, I sink into the all-too-familiar contours of the couch, pile the blankets on, and lie there shivering and crying. I'm taking perverse pleasure in this well of self-pity.

The Osprey Lakes Inn always serves lunch to all the slide-builders. I won't go this year. I haven't worked hard enough. I'm not hungry anyway. Crying hard, I squeeze my eyes shut, determined to be miserable. But cancer won't let things be that easy. All I have to do is wonder what the Inn will be serving. Just that mild bit of curiosity, and my mind lifts with a facility born of illness. I ponder my choices. What will be on the menu this year? That wonderful chili, thick with beans and an orchestra of spices? Or, perhaps it will be lasagna. There is no fuel like pasta. In my mind's eye, I experience the steamy warmth, fragrant with firewood and cooking, that greets the workers as they come through the door. The room is packed with people wolfing down platefuls of food, wiping the last morsels with crusty slices, going back for more, laughing, exchanging updates on the progress at the harvest and construction sites. Lunch is over too quickly. Smitty and his crew don't even pause for dessert but grab handfuls of chocolate chip cookies on their way out and back to work. A few of us always linger a bit too long, unable to pull ourselves away from the fire. I am so happy. The fire at the Inn merges dreamlike with the curling flames in my own living room. I drift off to sleep, nourished by all that glows around me.

I sleep through the rest of the slide-building. By the next morning, when I finally wander over to view the finished product, they are just getting ready to launch the first test ride. The experts who built the slide enthusiastically pile on the wooden toboggan for the first run, a safety check. Their very eagerness is testimony to the confidence and pride they have in their work. The year they choose to send a flatlander down first, I'm going to refuse to go anywhere near the slide for the entire season of operation.

Monday I get good news. My white count is moving in the right direction. They schedule me for my sixth and final chemotherapy treatment on the upcoming Friday. It's a mixed blessing. I dread the treatment, or at least I dread the two weeks following the treatment, but I still feel ready to rejoice. The end is in sight. If I can just survive this, soon it will all be behind me. January both begins and ends this year with an emphasis on purification rites. I think back to Venus in the morning sky and know I prefer that gentle centering to the chemical ordeal that is in store. However, I find it helpful to see this as purification rather than pollution. Friday, my body will be purged of any stray cancer cell resilient enough to have held on through the earlier treatments. I think there is going to be some celebrating in my future.

I was born February sixteenth. In the weeks before Valentine's Day in my seventh-grade year, whenever I entered a room, whispering friends would poke their elbows about and nudge each other to silence. They weren't always quick enough, and overheard snatches of conversation soon led me to understand that there was a party to which I had not been invited. I told myself it didn't matter, but for five nights running, I cried myself to sleep. One night Mother quietly entered the room and asked what was wrong. "Nothing," I lied, "sometimes I just like to cry."

The night of the party, Patsy Kelly called me in an apparent panic. Her dog had been hit by a car. Could I get my parents to drive me to her house so I could help her bandage and treat it? Because my nurturing response to anything furred or feathered was near legendary at school, it never occurred to me to ask her why she didn't call a veterinarian. Sandy, Gail, and I were always using eyedroppers to hand-raise the baby mice and rabbits disrupted by farm equipment. We often had a recuperating lamb or cat or raccoon in a box in some warm place in the house.

I bought the ruse without question. It was only on the way to Patsy's house that I remembered the party. I was stricken with embarrassment and dreaded walking in on all the fun from which I had so obviously been excluded. Not even the shouted "Surprise!"—not even the presents all bearing my name—convinced me it was really my party. It was only when I saw Patsy's dog jumping healthily about that I finally believed.

On the ride home, Mother brought up the subject of my tears and allowed that if she had thought I'd been crying because I hadn't been invited, she would have told me of the surprise. "Oh, no," I assured her, "that isn't why. Sometimes I just like to cry." My pain was still so real, however falsely conceived, that the comfort of my necessary lie assumed the status of truth.

Chapter 10

February

The days have steadily been lengthening since December 22, but only now do I notice the earlier onset of daybreak. Not until I moved to Osprey Lakes did I become aware of the wonderful complexities of light. Once the winter solstice passes, the days do, indeed, grow longer, but the bulk of the increase comes at the end of the day. Mornings remain stubbornly dark, with no apparent change until February. That first cherished light of February is a subtle, gentle increase. It isn't until March that light comes roaring at us with a grand explosion at either end of the day.

Unfortunately, the first Monday, Wednesday, and Friday of the month, Carol and I are running in dark even more serious than that offered up by January.

"You're a fool or a masochist," I tell her. "You could be wrapped in warm sheets sleeping."

"No, no," she lies. "I like to get up this early. I get more done. It gives me a start on the day."

We're out on the road an hour ahead of our usual schedule. We're in the homestretch following my last chemotherapy treatment. Today I'll head back in to the hospital for eight hours of IV fluids and Zofran. Knowing I'll get to spend the day sleeping in the chemo room makes it easier for me to get up so early. I don't know what Carol tells herself. Once again, she is an awfully good sport, an awfully good friend. She never lets me run alone, always claims some change in her own schedule that requires her to arise just as early as I must.

The snow is so cold we have trouble hearing each other over the squeak squeak our feet make as they pack last night's two inches into the hard base already covering the road. I am feeling lousy. "There's lead poisoning. There's mercury poisoning. And there's platinum poisoning," I tell her. "Platinum is definitely the blue-chip commodity." She has heard my routine before. It is something more than nausea that wears me down. I squirm with a deep bodily unease, a sense that some leaching toxin has invaded every pore. Strangely enough, running helps. I play all kind of head games with myself, am convinced that the exercise opens the capillaries up, forces the killer chemicals into the deepest recess of my bowels, ferrets out the stray cancer cell hiding almost out of reach. I tell myself that it's a two-stage process. First the running forces the cisplatin through my body, then it flushes it out.

There is something almost celebratory in my complaints. I give in with a vengeance to the urge to whine. This is almost over. I can let go of my stiff upper lip. I'm allowed to truly hate this, because I'm not going to have to do it anymore. I know from experience, if I can just get through the next ten days, I'll get to recover without being knocked down again.

"Just hang on for another week," Carol tells me. Suddenly, I feel sad. I don't think Carol ever wanted to learn this much about cancer. I didn't either, and yet the experience has been a good one for me. Much as I complain, I wouldn't want to go back to my precancer state. I say that all the time. I think I mean it even if I eventually die of this disease. Everybody dies sometime. If cancer was going to make me die while the rest of the world got to live, I'd be really furious. But everybody dies, and I wouldn't want to do so without the insights that have been cancer's gift. But what about Carol? She suffers through all the downsides, but can't possibly be seized by the joy that is mine in those unexpected moments when clarity descends and lifts me away from physical restraints. I decide that illness is much harder for those who watch than it is for those embraced by disease.

"A lovely thing this cancer." We laugh. "You know," I continue, "it never was the disease that made me sick. Only the treatments." As I say the words, I realize I am talking in the past tense.

I finish the run holding my breath, crossing my fingers. I have cut myself loose from this disease. I am on my own. Am I brave enough to live without the crutch my illness has become? I hesitate. There is still the final CAT scan. The doctors won't officially end the treatments, there will be no diplomas issued, until I successfully navigate that medical graduation ceremony.

Each year I forget about February. Oh, I can talk about it. I intellectualize. I verbalize. I can describe what happens in February, but even so I am unprepared for the effect of the shift in light that is, for me, more uplifting in February than in any other month of the year. My daughter Ingrid's birthday is February fifth. It is always around that time that the first impossible blue captures the sky. Blue, blue, February blue. Only September comes close to rivaling that shade. If I could cut just a swatch from the dome of sky in each of those months and lay the pieces side by side away from all else, I think it possible that I could not tell one from the other. But September, uncut, has all the distraction of turning leaves, late-blooming flowers. February has only white snow. All those rays of light are bounced back into the sky, deepened, intensified, distilled into blue so pure the eye is almost unable to comprehend its full richness.

There is a certain slant of light in February that writes spring across even the most frozen ground. Until that happens, I have forgotten that I even want April. The months of deep winter are all about survival. Perhaps I am made senseless with cold, so burdened with resignation, so preoccupied with mere endurance that I allow no flirtation with thoughts of green leaves, warm breezes. And then the light changes in February, and my blood rises with the sap. I anticipate some sweetness. When I was young and pulled by this cosmic promise, I was sure that I was about to fall in love. Because I pinned my hopes on the substantial, I was invariably disappointed. It has taken me all these years to learn that what I felt was already love. Love is not something that happens. It requires no subject, no object. It simply is, and nothing evokes its heady buoyancy for me as much as being carried on the cusp between changing seasons.

February sunrises are like the inside of a seashell, all silvered pearl with pale streaks of lavender, pink, and topaz. I love it when the air is so cold that any hint of moisture freezes into floating dust of frost. In the early mornings this coats even the smallest twig with glitter that reflects and sparkles in anticipation of the brighter light to come. A similar phenomenon works on the steamy breath that Carol, Chuckles, and I spew forth as we chug up and down these hills at dawn. The resulting hoarfrost transforms Chuckles in a particularly spectacular fashion. It doesn't happen on our afternoon walks. I think it takes some combination of the early-morning cold and the hot, deep breath inspired by his vigorous trot.

I have never owned a dog I didn't see as absolutely beautiful. I suspect that love coats the lenses of my eyes, because rarely do others reinforce my judgment. In fact, our dear old Scoobie, a mixed breed whose pedigree was quite short on both sides, was most often compared by strangers to Cujo, of Stephen King fame. I told myself that these were just people who were afraid of dogs. Even my children, who loved Scoobie as much as I did, howled with laughter when I flipped through the newest batch of photographs and asked in dismay, "How come I can never get a good picture of Scoobie?" Apparently, it takes the flesh-and-blood creature to fog my eyes.

However, Chuckles is so truly magnificent that even a total stranger will be moved to exclaim, "That is the most beautiful dog I have ever seen." (In the beginning, when he was a puppy and I was still mourning Scoobie, this hurt my feelings. "How come nobody ever told me Scoobie was beautiful?" I would ask myself.) To the uninitiated, Chuckles looks like an ebony version of a golden retriever. If I had ever seen a flat-coat before we purchased Chuckles, I would have assumed it was a cross between a black lab and a golden. Chuckles weighs about eighty-five pounds. All the exercise has resulted in a proud, strong carriage that telegraphs joy and confidence. His coat is so shiny that people are always asking what we feed him. If I thought the luster could be attributed to diet alone, I would join him in his bowl of Pro Plan and brewer's yeast. In fact, the glossy coat is considered a breed characteristic.

Now on this particular February morning, the tips of all the fur within reach of his steaming breath are frosted white. Each whisker, each eyelash, bears testimony to the minus twelve degrees registered on the thermometer. Chuckles has a mane of hair around his neck that continues to the wavy V of feathers that adorns his prominent chest. Each wave is accented in white. Even his shoulders and the long coat flowing from his front legs are coated in frost. I look to Carol for confirmation of his beauty and discover that she is similarly decorated. The hair that escapes from her hat is fringed with frost as are her eyelashes and eyebrows. At the corners of her eyes, the upper and lower lashes are freezing together. "You should see yourself," I tell her.

"You too," she responds. I may not have much hair left, but it still constitutes a headful, however sparse. I put my hand up to touch the few short strands that curl around the edges of my cap. They are stiff with ice. However, I understand that since every remaining hair on my head is now pure white of its own accord, no one but Carol could possibly notice. My eyelashes and eyebrows disappeared months ago. So we run in descending orders of contrast. My frost offers no change from the usual condition. Carol's is subtle, like the work of a skilled beautician. And Chuckles is a whole new parti-colored dog, spectacular in his display of the whitest white against the blackest black.

It is not just the light that changes in February. There are a host of other signs of impending spring. The last thing I hear before falling off to sleep at night is the soft, mournful call of the great horned owl. And, if I'm lucky, the same deep hoot pulls me from sleep before the alarm has a chance to go off. Frank, our postmaster and deputy game warden, once explained that this is a mating call. In those early-morning hours, I sometimes wonder what owlish wisdom has tinged love's song with melancholy. But now, Frank entertains me with tales of a favorite February sport, "hooting in the owls." After work, he and his two boys stand in their backyard mimicking the three-note cry and counting the number of owls they can call in on a given evening. Luckily, this human subterfuge is only temporarily successful. By the end of the month, these winged creatures of the night will all have found appropriate owl companions and will already be on the nest, incubating eggs in temperatures that are often well below freezing.

I am surprised at the amount of anxiety engendered by the schedule that arrives from Geisinger confirming my CAT scan appointment. I'm due in there on the twenty-sixth of the month. So, we will soon find out if I've been kidding myself with all those visualizations picturing an intestine and diaphragm completely free of tumors. Fortunately, this hospital generally does not perform "look/see" surgery following treatment for ovarian cancer. The rationale makes sense to me. Tiny new-growth tumors might be missed even with surgery. The doctors are willing to put their faith in the combined diagnostic of the CA 125 and the CAT scan. That suits me just fine. I am not in the mood for the trauma of another major surgery. The last one is still too fresh in my mind.

The night before my appointment, Chuckles and I have a lovely walk. Gene is still in Philadelphia. He'll be up tonight and will go to the hospital with me for moral support. I've been tough about not letting him accompany me when I go for chemo. Ever since his comment about doctors playing games of hide-and-seek, I've been convinced that the eight-hour stretch goes by more easily for me when I don't have to worry about how someone else is handling it and can simply concentrate on myself. Cancer has made me selfish. But tomorrow I do want Gene there. I'm planning on a celebration. I push any other thoughts away, let them just trail off unfinished.

Chuckles pulls me back to the here and now as he dives through the snow after a rabbit. He has never caught one on the run, but he surely does glory in the chase. What little I know about Eastern religions convinces me that dogs have much to teach us. If being fully present is a sign of enlightenment, then Chuckles is my model. He exists totally in each moment and always with joy. "The thing I love most about Chuckles is how happy he is," I once told Ingrid.

"And what in the world could he possibly find to be *unhappy* about?" Ingrid teases me over how we spoil this pup, and, indeed, he has the perfect life for a dog bred to the field and human companionship. He is always at my side. After Scoobie's death, I vowed I would never get another dog. Their life spans are too short, and I intended not to allow myself to be that vulnerable to pain. Ingrid was dismayed. "You have to get another dog. Osprey Lakes is the ideal spot. It's not fair to deprive some dog of the life you offer here."

I whistle and he bounds back to me. Reaching down, I pat his head. If I pull through this, I will owe much to my loyal four-footed companion. With Gene still working three days a week and gone so much, I had no choice but to get Chuckles out for his exercise every day. I always felt better at the end of the two-mile loop around the Laurel Path than I had at the beginning.

The snow is still fairly deep, but the blackened bark of the trees has absorbed the sun's heat. At the base of each trunk, the snow has been sculpted away, shrinking back from the captured warmth, making room for the life evidenced by this first visible sign. We've passed the beach and are heading home. This east side has always been my favorite. The path has more tangled roots stretching across it. There are powerful rock formations to scramble over and around. Perhaps because the walking is more difficult, one encounters fewer people here, even in the summer months. Today we are utterly alone. Not until the weekend operation of the slide draws visitors to us will our lake evidence much sign of human habitation. During the week, the only human footprints I encounter are my own.

As we approach Lovers' Leap Rock, Chuckles suddenly freezes, and all the hair goes up on his back. I reach down and grab his collar at the same time that I follow his gaze to the hemlock just ahead of us on the path. One of the previous year's bear cubs has been pulled out of his den by the warm sun. At the sound of our approach, he is rapidly backing down the tree, a compact furry bundle that probably weighs less than Chuckles. The cub hits the ground in a roll and just continues tumbling until he disappears into one of the many small caves that network this area. We race over to look for some sign of him, some footprint that I can offer as proof, but the only evidence of his passing is a flattened place in the snow that won't survive the evening's blowing drifts. Chuckles races excitedly about. However, with perhaps more wisdom than I possess, he is not as eager as I am to peer into the hole that swallowed our fat friend. Bears are not true hibernators. Even in January, they will come out if the weather warms. Still, I have never seen a bear in winter before and consider this sighting a happy omen.

Gene has left work early and is at the house when Chuckles and I return. We are all sorry that he wasn't with us to see the bear. But it is nice to have something so exciting to share, and I am happy that there is a topic other than CAT scans to occupy our conversation.

I retire to my bedroom early, still sleeping in my own room. I wonder if cancer will ever release its jealous hold. All my energy is concentrated in the fight. I struggle to keep some identity that is truly mine. There is a funny contradiction here. I have been shameless about sharing the experience with family and friends, but much as I reveal, there is still some part of my core that is walled off. Some piece of me needs to travel this alone.

I have a great deal of difficulty falling asleep. I lie there for a long time, trying the meditation that has been so helpful the past nine or ten months. Nothing works. Has all my brave talk been a sham? "Will this intense joy at simply being alive ever fade?" I asked in our Christmas letter. "One of the best things about having had cancer is that I now know absolutely that I will someday die. Of course, everyone understands this intellectually. But I experience the knowledge with a certainty that feels like comfort. As a result, I have this wonderful sense of being a tourist in the world—all the heightened awareness and excitement that comes with travel to exotic places, only I get to sleep in a predictably familiar bed every night."

What a hypocrite I am. If this anxiety is not fear of death, fear of disease, what is it? It is easy to be comfortable with dying pushed off into the nameless future. It would appear that I am not so good with dying that could happen in the next few months, even the next year or two. I finally fall asleep crying, mostly, I think, for the loss of the graceful faith that has so often enabled me to experience the spherical union of life and death. But the unity for me is broken, and tonight the lovely three-dimensional orb has been pounded into a flat oppositional coin. Life on one side. Death on the other. Heads I win. Tails I lose.

Long before morning, long before my alarm goes off, I am awakened by an abundance of light. I am filled with light. It expands, and I expand with it. My boundaries dissolve in the presence of full-spectrum white. Never have I longed to be so fully possessed by anything. I float in a room without walls, afraid to open my eyes, afraid to breathe. I don't want to move for fear something will dislodge this splendor. Observe, I wordlessly tell myself. Observe. Notice. Watch. It does not go away. I forget caution and give in to wonder. The light is dazzling. However, it does not blind, but illuminates. Oh, that dust of morning frost is nothing to this densely packed iridescent glory. This is the brightest incandescence I have ever experienced, but I can gaze directly at it with no visual pain. My eyes remain closed; this is not something to see in the conventional sense. It is something that fills me, that surrounds and supports me. I am suffused with light. I am possessed by light. I am carried by light, transported with joy. At last I simply sink back into it. I feel my head tilt, tumbling backward into comfort so profound that there is no question and no need for answer. I sleep as I have never slept before.

When the alarm goes off, I wake up almost unwilling to move. I don't want anything to shake me loose from the night's radiance. Something profound has happened that really can't be captured by conventional language. Later, I will tell. Later still I will write these words, knowing even as I tell, even as I write, that this won't be believed. The obvious charge will be that I was dreaming. However, I know that this was no dream. It feels like the most authentically real event of my life. I am not a traditionally religious person. But it's funny how I have learned the art of faith. I have learned to accept without questioning that for which there is no rational explanation. To force reason on this experience requires a faith in reason's power that is as without claim to proof as is the faith that enables me simply to accept the experience, no questions asked. I was raised a Quaker, but in recent years I have not even gone to meeting. My spiritual sense has always felt more confined than expanded by religious doctrine. Quakers believe that no person outside oneself can serve as the interpreter of God. There is a bit of God in every person. Listen to the inner light. Let that light be your source of truth. The night's occurrence was not a revelation for me in the sense that I now know something withheld from me before. My answer to all the big questions remains "I don't know." The night was simply a gift, magnificent, though brief. I have no wisdom, only gratitude and wonder.

I am quiet on the drive to the hospital, but I don't feel afraid. Before long, however, the only reality is hospital routine. I truly hate CAT scans. A medical intern brings the heavy-ion cocktail that, given time, will illuminate my intestines. He leaves me with two glasses of the chalky substance. One to drink now, one at ten-thirty. "It's kind of like a milk shake." Oh, right. I have been this route before, and if I could truly believe the milk shake line, I would forswear butterfat forever. Unfortunately for my figure, my passion for chocolate malteds remains even after hearing this vile concoction called a milk shake. Gene and I make small talk. We watch the clock. I am a tough case. Not even last night's serenity can push back the little claws of fear scratching at my attempts at composure. Finally, it's my turn. I strip and don the hospital gown. Even as they tell me which is front and which is back, I forget. I have never acquired hospital fashion sense. The room is cold. The technician packs warmed cotton blankets around me. He starts the procedure: tip this way, roll that way, move that chalk into all the loops and turns. I try hard to be a model patient, want nothing to mask the truth that lies within. Finally we are ready and the cameras start their slow path down my torso. I begin shaking violently. He can't take the pictures until I stop. But this shaking is sort of like suppressed childhood giggles. The meaner the teacher, the more difficult it is to get them under control. "I think we need more hot blankets," he tells me.

No warmth in the world is going to work on this case of the shakes. "You know," I confess after I have been packed with all the blankets he can crowd around me, "I think I'm just scared. Blankets aren't going to do much for that." Foolishly, I start to cry. "The only other CAT scan I've had was when they discovered my cancer." He hands me some paper tissues. "The technician called the surgeon in. He stood right where you're standing and told me I was a mass of tumors, probably ovarian in origin. I think I'm just afraid." Confession must be good for the soul. Or else our conversation gives the blankets time to work their magic. I finally stop shaking, and we get on with it. This time there is no retracing of steps, no going back for second shots, no long pauses to go to the phone and place a call. I'm feeling brave, pretty confident. "Does it look good?" I ask him. "Do you think I'm clean?"

He helps me up. "I can't answer that. Your doctor will read these pictures and talk to you about it."

As Gene and I leave the waiting room, we see Dr. Silverman scurrying in one of the side doors to X ray. His presence sends a chill. "That's a bad sign," I tell my husband. "He shouldn't be up here now. He read my MRIs downstairs. I don't think he should be coming up here now. That's a bad sign."

"Well, aren't MRIs and CAT scans different things?" Gene's trying for comfort, but logic can't touch my apprehensions. Besides he is intimidated by the human body. He is a city boy and has always quickly backed down in any discussion that even touches on biology. When we were first married, I listened in astonishment as he, in all seriousness, explained to Dana, his fourteen-year-old daughter, that when dogs mate in the winter, they freeze together and must be thawed apart by throwing buckets of cold water on them. I interjected by telling them both more of the details of dog copulation than any teenage girl—or her father—could possibly have wanted to know.

Since then, Gene has meekly taken my word on all things biological. I've spent a lot of time in Geisinger's medical library checking out the survival rates achieved by various approaches to ovarian cancer. My first visits were inspired by confrontations in which I tried in vain to get Dr. Silverman to lower the dosage of carboplatin he was giving me. I never did go back and apologize for being so stubborn, but the more I read, the more faith I had in this man's chemical wizardry. I remind myself of that now. My treatment has been cutting edge. If anyone can beat this devil in my belly, it will be Dr. Silverman. Dr. Silverman, red-clover-blossom tea, and February light.

We have time to kill, but I don't want any lunch. I play with a bowl of lentil soup while Gene goes for the lasagna. We read or pretend to read. We browse the hospital gift shop. We wander through the halls. Finally, it is close to my appointed hour with the man who already knows my fate, and we go down to the ground floor to hang out in the oncology waiting room. The nurses here are unbelievably warm. How do they remember everyone's name? How do they stay so universally cheerful? I recall my first visit here, the skepticism I felt when obviously familiar patients came in laughing and joking with the staff. "Some denial going on there," I had smugly told myself. Now I'm the one who laughs and jokes. We're still here, aren't we? That's the lesson. It's not cancer that kills us, it's time. Mortality is not restricted to cancer patients. But today, it's time I bargain for.

Debbie flips through my records. "Big day. You had your CAT scan. He'll see you soon." I struggle to read her face, then decide she doesn't know. No point putting her on the spot by asking. Lots of folks come over and chat with me. Strange how much I love this place. I feel supported by a roomful of friends. Then Dr. Silverman comes out to bring some papers to the desk. I try to catch his eye. Once we stopped fighting, he has always greeted me warmly. Today, he won't even look in my direction. "A bad sign," I tell Gene. "That's a bad sign. He didn't even say hi."

"I don't think he saw you," Gene reassures me.

I'm not buying comfort that cheap. "No. I know he saw me. He just wouldn't look. That's a bad sign."

I, who have been steadfast in my belief in the value of a positive attitude, today will not allow myself one shred of hope that could prove to be false. The chips are down. I steel myself against any disappointment. At last Linda calls my name. Dr. Silverman is pulling my files from the slot outside the examining room. He gives me a big smile. "It looks good." I am incredulous, want to make sure I've heard him right. I cover my gaping mouth with both hands, actually gasping for breath. "There are no signs of tumors on your CAT scan."

"Gene," I call.

Linda is smiling happily. "Do you want me to go get him for you?"

The mood is celebratory. I want everyone to know, but Linda and Dr. Silverman move us toward the examining room. I am aware that perhaps there are others for whom the news has not been as happy. "Heather is gloating," one of the other nurses teases. She is right. I am, but I want everyone to believe that this can happen to them too. I feel like running through the chemo room like a crazed cheerleader, calling out to those pinned there by slowly dripping IVs that they should love the drugs that scar their veins and steal their hair and turn them inside out with nausea. I want to tell them that it all passes. That this too will someday end. But the staff have seen too many endings other than the one we celebrate in this small room and wisely keep me here.

Dr. Silverman is explaining as he always does—thoroughly, technically. For once, I can't hold to every word. I'm lost in the big picture. My cancer is gone. I hear some of it. "If we still did look/see surgery and the surgery confirmed what the CAT scan shows, it would mean that you now have a sixty percent chance that your tumors will not return. Forty percent of the women who are clean at the end of treatment will someday have a recurrence." Sixty percent might as well be 100 percent as far as I'm concerned. There's just enough doubt in there to keep me humble, fully alive. Since the very beginning, every cut of the deck has placed me in the lucky half. I've come a long way since I pushed a young intern into talking odds with me. "Not good," she'd said. "Not good." I pressed her, preparing myself for 1 or 2 percent. After all, anyone I'd ever known with ovarian cancer had died. She finally answered. "Less than ten percent."

She must have thought me mad. "Ten percent!" I whooped. "Those are terrific odds." I arrogantly added, "I'm used to living in the ninety-seventh percentile."

Sixty percent has a friendly, reassuring sound. Right now, today, I'm cancer free. That's all that counts with me. That's all any healthy person can say. I'm solidly in the ranks of the living. *No one* knows what tomorrow will bring. I'm just like anybody else. As we're leaving, I ask Dr. Silverman the question I didn't have the courage to ask until now. "What would have happened if the tumors had still been there? What would the next step have been?"

"We'd have waited a little while, given you a rest, and then started in with chemotherapy again."

Gene and I float out of the hospital. He races ahead and starts dropping quarters in the pay phone. He dials Ingrid. Then Craig. We call all the kids. Lots of laughter, tears, relieved rejoicing. "Do you want to go somewhere to celebrate?" Gene asks me.

I shake my head. "Just home. I want to see Chuckles. And Carol. Can we stop and get her some flowers? She has been more loyal and forgiving than anyone ought to have to be. I know she's home chewing her nails, waiting to see how all this has turned out."

Soon after we get home, the FTD man shows up with a huge bouquet of pink roses from Ingrid. When I call, she confesses that she had ordered them days before. "To celebrate you being in the pink." She laughs. "I was pretty confident, but you'll notice I didn't put that on the card, just in case . . ."

There is nothing more fun than spreading good news. We end the month joyfully praising the normal life. I put a sign up in the post office, thanking everyone but mostly letting them know that all those casseroles can start going to other people.

I've always felt close to trees. When I was an adolescent, my surface awkward-ness disguised a wild inner union with the natural world. I remember waking one May night and creeping barefoot through the sleeping house, drawn outside by some magnetic pull. Behind the old chicken coop, one twisted survivor of what was once an apple orchard glowed white and fragrant with improbable blossom. The ancient tree had not borne fruit during our somewhat brief tenure on the property, and I had no reason to believe the present year would be any different. Something about the persistent push for life in defiance of the inevitability of ruin and decay made me unaccountably sad. I remember throwing my arms around the tree and hugging it until the rough bark scratched painfully into my cheek. I pressed harder still. I wanted to be scarred by that tree. If I could just clasp it tightly enough to break the surface tension, I felt I would lose all boundaries, become the tree, be-come the night vapors, the farthest distant star. But I remained girl and tree re-mained tree, and at last, feeling slightly chastised and foolish, I returned to bed.

Chapter 11

March

In Osprey Lakes, March and April are lumped together without affection as mud season. But, of course, part of March's charm is its unpredictability. Here on the mountain, it goes out like a lion as often as it comes in like one. The worst winter storm in our years in Sullivan County occurred on March 13. Spring flirts, but it is best not to take her promises seriously. At least not if it is warm weather that defines the season for you. The reputation for mud seems a bit undeserved or at least overstated, and I suspect it to be a local ploy to discourage the snowbirds, those retired residents heading back from Florida, from landing much before June.

By the time March rolls around, I am always restive, pushing for change of some undefined type. Even my body feels locked into repetitive rhythms that fail to comfort and leave me feeling bored and annoyed. I crave something different. One year, March obliged by surprising Carol and me with the best cross-country skiing of the season. That glorious March, we broke completely from our ritualized runs and skied instead. The old railroad bed cuts through the forest and catches very little late-day sun. As long as we were out there by 7 A.M., the trail was frozen hard and fast. It was marvelous. With each fresh snowfall, we carefully cut new tracks on the old base. Since the afternoon sun kept the snow melted from most lawns, no one else thought of skiing and the track was custom-made for our skis and width of stride. I remember with joy the animal enthusiasm with which we attacked the course. We did it as an out-and-back sprint, pushing hard from the Outlet Pond through the woods until we hit the open fields that signaled the approach to the park.

When we reached the park, we would change lead and race back for the Outlet Pond. We did these early-morning skis as workouts. Invariably, we dressed too warmly and would fling jackets, caps, gloves, and scarves off as we raced along. I can't speak for Carol, but I imbued each workout with a level of competition totally absent from our morning runs. When we run, we talk nonstop. It is a time for sharing gossip, banalities, dreams, frustrations, pithy insights on the never-ending war between the sexes, and humor. One of the women in town who walks the lake counterclockwise each morning at about the same time we do our clockwise jaunt cornered us at the spaghetti dinner. "I'm so impressed with the fact that you two are always talking when I see you." I thought she was making reference to our superior conditioning and could feel myself puffing with pride at our ability to talk while we sped along. However, Rita quickly set me straight. "You see each other every morning. Don't you ever run out of things to say?"

Our morning runs may be about sisterhood, but those March skiing work-outs were about strength and speed. I'm not a naturally athletic person. My only real skill is stubbornness. What I lack in ability, I make up for in deter-mination. Back in the days when I ran marathons, I was known as the bad-weather animal. The worse the conditions, the higher my respective placing in the race. Give me a hilly cross-country trail that is rutted and strewn with rocks, roots, and dry washes, and I'll finish somewhere in the money. My best placing in a half marathon was in a race that foolishly went off despite hur-ricane conditions. Dogged determination is my strong suit. I never was fast. The longer the race, the higher my placing. In my running prime, long since behind me, Gene used to tell people that if he pushed me off a building, I would fall at a steady eight minutes a mile.

My family has always joked that I will race anything that doesn't know it is in a race. I wish I could declare the observation false, but there is an un-pleasant truth to it. Those of us who are born with the curse of a competi-tive spirit locked in a no-talent body must take our wins where we can fashion them. When we lived in center-city Philadelphia, I got around on a beat-up one-speed bike that was my pride and joy. Wonder Bike. On it, I was certain

I could leap over tall buildings in a single bound. Many was the fish delivery truck I left in my wake. What Wonder Bike and I lacked in speed, we made up for in a reckless ability to maneuver through tight spots and a willingness to challenge yellow turning fast to red. In retrospect, I know I was a hazard and don't recommend the sport of racing fish trucks. Tugboats are a safer venture. Gene and I used to run together on the piers at Penn's Landing. He claims that when he suddenly found me picking up speed, he knew to look out into the river for a tugboat that I almost certainly was racing to the end of the wharf.

Did Carol know that March that she was in a race? I've never asked her. I do know that I always waited to toss my shed garments until there was a bush that would hold them within arm's reach for me on the way back, so determined was I not to lose a split second stooping to retrieve a sweaty pair of gloves. How can one race on a course that is designed to be single file and contains an automatic change of lead at the halfway mark? The beauty of unilaterally declared competitions is that one can structure the rules to guarantee success. I counted it a win if I managed to decrease the distance between Carol and me from start to finish whenever she headed out first. I was likewise victorious if I increased the distance when I was breaking trail. Did I end the spring skiing season a champion? The fact that I can't recall would indicate that I did not. However, I am safe in saying that it was glorious good fun for both of us. We always ended the sprint breathless and laughing, finding in that push for speed just the change we needed to carry us happily through the last days of winter.

I have not been skiing at all this year. Winter is almost over, and I know that my skis will remain untouched, propped against the basement wall. And this has been a wonderful year for snow, a true Osprey Lakes winter. The snow that started in November has just been building ever since. It's an almost imperceptible thing, a steady accumulation, just enough of a dusting every night to keep things magically fresh, no gray, discolored snow for Osprey Lakes, not even this late in the season. I have a friend who continued to cross-country ski despite treatment for a brain tumor. I admire Red's tenacity and courage and wonder if my old competitive spirit has been lost somewhere over the long haul of these past few months. Running is something I do almost on automatic pilot. It's as much a part of my morning ritual as brushing my teeth. For the past eighteen years my day has begun with a morning run. I don't know how *not* to run. But I do know how not to ski, and although I look longingly at the perfect conditions, at the first thought of clamping down the bindings, I feel crushed by a bone-deep weariness. Next year, I tell myself.

Those who need warmth to herald spring are bound to be disappointed by March. But for those of us content with other offerings, March has delights indeed. I am a person who finds most rodents cute. Since I have never witnessed a rat in Osprey Lakes, I can nearly claim to find *all* rodents cute. However, the absolute best in a category already defined by bright-eyed appeal is the chipmunk. Each year I spot the first one of the season in some quick tail-flicking moment just between the last month of official winter and the first one of spring. I regret that Spike, our cat, is as drawn to them as I am but with a very different conclusion in mind. Luckily, as Spike heads into his fifteenth year, he is less often seen with the tip of a small tail poking toothpick fashion from the corner of his mouth. He will have to content himself with joining me in chipmunk *watching*.

Osprey Lakes has a huge chipmunk population. All the old Victorian stone walls provide wonderful hiding and nesting places. I will ever be in awe of the miracle of nature that produces those precision stripes, in lovely shades of black and tawny brown, around each eye, down each trim little back. March's first chipmunks are mostly seen skittering across the crust of snow at the base of our bird feeder. Chipmunks have a feature that the red and the gray squirrels, adorable though they be, completely lack: cheek pouches. A chipmunk will stuff these full of sunflower seeds until the bulges reach partway down his back. Looking like someone long overdue for a root canal, he staggers about almost thrown out of balance by his greed. Later in the summer, I will sit on our screened porch and watch families of four to six babies engage in endless games of chase and tag. It seems to be good chipmunk form for the youngster "tagged" to leap straight up into the air upon

contact. We have a rotting woodpile in our side yard that I won't allow anyone to tidy up, as it is a favorite chipmunk playground.

Birdsong also changes in March. We hear the cardinals much more frequently and melodiously. I heard my first song sparrow this morning and
later in the day spotted a pair of them flitting in the lower branches of the old
rhododendron bushes in front of the house. Lacking an ear for music, I can
distinguish by their calls only the most common birds. I just know that the
air is filled with sweeter sound in March, a phenomenon that will continue
building to a symphonic climax in May.

Close to the ground, January and February are white, gray, and silver
months. March brings a lovely red cast to the tips of roadside shrubs. Color
surfaces everywhere. The goldfinch begins to lose the soft olive that has let
him move incognito through the winter. Most of the males now sport hints
of the yellow that will blaze to full golden glory in the summer months.

March is skunk month. I am one who finds the musky aroma of skunk intoxicating, and I rejoice each year in that pungent odor as a sure sign of
spring. March must be their mating season, because suddenly the scent of
them is everywhere. Chuckles, amazingly enough for a dog that spends as
much time outside as he does, has never tangled with a skunk. For this I am
grateful, because skunk smell is not nearly so pleasant when confronted up
close in the full intensity of a dog that has been sprayed. I once had a springer
spaniel that would not leave skunks alone. I think the first one that hit her
made her so mad that she declared a lifelong war on them. It was a war that
she consistently lost. Forget what they say about tomato juice, forget what
they say about toothpaste. The only thing that I have ever found to work at
removing the evidence of a dog/skunk encounter is time. And even then,
damp days bring the memory persistently back.

Near the end of this changeling month where I can go to bed in one season
and wake in another, I begin to feel some changes of my own. My life is coming back as surely as the migratory birds. My white counts still aren't up
where anyone wants them to be, but I feel health pushing through the fading remnants of chemical treatment in the same way that the bulbs Dee and

I planted last October form heaped mounds under the crust of winter. No spear of green has yet broken the surface, but doesn't the earth feel the movement? And so I can feel my own life return before signs are visible even to those who search the neatly labeled vials of my blood.

I believe I have defeated cancer, but I know that I will not defeat death. Nor do I any longer wish to. Life and death are all tangled up inside me. It is easier for me now to cross the divide and hold, for just a moment, brief union with trees. March in Sullivan County is maple syrup month. Even here the world has gone too high-tech for wooden buckets and spouts tapped into trees, but as I drive by a maple grove, not even the plastic collecting lines looping through the woods can distance me from the sense that the sap that flows there is drawn from my own blood.

The sadness I felt as a child, the sadness to which beauty can inspire me still, is the tender melancholy of separation. I used to believe that the purpose of death was to make us appreciate life. My encounter with cancer has knocked that perception off a bit. I am very aware of the burdens of physical life. The body, at best, is a failing thing. Illness has led me to understand the weight of movement. Even that which we celebrate, food and feasting, is not a voluntary ritual but a harsh necessity masquerading as banquet. Existence in this physical world requires tremendous effort. It is hard work. Sometimes when my meditations took me skimming on ocean surface, breaking occasionally even with that and lifting into the void, free of material definition, I sensed the joy in the loss of life's shackles. I now believe that the purpose of life is to help us appreciate death. How grand a thing when all beauty is mine, when no physical boundary stands between me and the sunrise, the first pale anemone translucent against leaf mold and moss. The sadness I felt at the distance between me and apple blossoms will evaporate when all is one.

For now, however, I remain firmly attached to material existence. I think the faces of my grandchildren hold me here. Each one so excellent in its uniqueness. I marvel at the curve of a forehead, the sweet perfection of fringed eyelashes dusting against plump cheeks. I adore the way their little mouths shape softly around the final *o* of their pet name for me, Baboo. What if I had no grandchildren? My children, grown or not, would be enough. What if I had no children? I would still stand amazed at the sight of a drifting osprey silhouetted against an impossibly blue sky. The truth is, I may not be afraid of death, but I certainly am not ready to die. There is too much to anchor me here with joy. Is this the dilemma that kept me awake the night before my CAT scan, not a fear of death so much as an awesome connection to life? Is anyone ever really ready to die? When I am 102, will I still find some attachment too strong to break? Or will the increasing burden of a failing body finally enable me to say a fond farewell to this physical existence? Only time will tell, and suddenly it is time I seem to have.

Anyone who loves weather as much as I do is bound to love March. Osprey Lakes is famous for its fog. When I was substitute teaching in Laporte, the town just five miles east of us, I could leave school under bright skies only to run smack into a home-based fog so thick that I could have walked as fast as I was willing to drive. In our first year in Sullivan County, I was so startled by the uniqueness of the climate zone in Osprey Lakes that I dubbed our newfound paradise Brigadoon. The weather would be clear in Muncy Valley, but halfway up the mountain, we would encounter a thick bank of fog. We don't get much fog in the winter months, but it returns like a seasonal bird when March arrives. March fog comes in different varieties. The wisdom among the toboggan slide builders is that fog will melt the ice more quickly than rain will. And certainly that has been true this year. After three days of heavy fog early in the month, the slide lay pitted and unstable and was closed for the season.

Last week, the fog moved in at about four in the afternoon. Gene and I walked Chuckles late that day. Despite the fog, the temperature was dropping as we made our way around the lake. Some magic alchemy combined cold and fog and transformed the woodlands as we watched. By the time we got back to the house, no twig or blade of dried grass was left uncoated by hoarfrost. Every single branch was outlined. The tiny ice crystals had a special affinity for the needles of the white pine. The frost dripped off them in dazzling chains. It's hard to imagine miniaturized snowflakes so tiny that they could etch each individual spine of a burdock, but they had indeed made a photo negative of the forest. What had been dark was now light. The precision of the pen that sketched the lines was flawless.

This morning, Chuckles and I stepped out to meet Carol in a world socked in by a heavy gray mist. This is a true spring fog, warm, moist, alive with something undefined. This is ice-melting, winter-chasing fog. As is so often the case with an unpredicted weather pattern, it has blown in from somewhere off the usual course, bringing with it a variety of birds. I can hear them in the treetops, flocks of them calling to each other, but the fog is too thick for me to make positive identification from their shadowy, flitting forms. They move about a bit like starlings but lack a starling's rasping call. The slightly quavering monotones make me want to say cedar waxwing, but it seems far too early for their return. I usually spot the first of those in June. I tend to see what it is I want to see. Waxwings are a special favorite on a list that puts starlings near the bottom. My safest call is none at all. Something wonderful in the trees is what I tell Carol when we connect up on the back side of the lake. And something wonderful on the lake, but there is no mystery here, Canadian geese, our most common harbingers of spring.

Carol and I can't see through the fog to the lake, but it is obvious from the commotion that a sizable flock of geese has touched down there. The lake is still frozen, or at least it was the last time we could see it, but this doesn't stop the geese. They light down as easily as they do on a newly planted cornfield. I remind Carol of the experience she had a few years ago under similar conditions. I was off the mountain for some reason and she was jogging alone. She was running on the road in a heavy fog, heading toward the beach. Just before she got there, a big, old bobcat sauntered out, crossing the road directly in front of her. He paid her almost no mind. He was obviously on his way to the lake to pick himself some breakfast from the honking, fog-shrouded throng. In our years here, Gene and I have on four occasions spotted bobcats from the car, but I have never seen one nose to nose. "I wish we'd see a bobcat now," I tell her, still impressed with the wonder of her lovely sighting.

"We won't. Rita could tell us why." We both laugh and say in unison, "We talk too much."

The local enthusiasm for geese is in exact proportion to their migratory reliability. They don't stay in Osprey Lakes long. They come through in early spring and again in fall, but their visits here are brief. So we don't suffer the goose-soiled beaches and parks so familiar to city folk. In a wild area, geese know how to behave like wild creatures. Two years ago, one brave pair stayed on in the Outlet Pond, managing to hatch just one fuzzy gosling, which grew into a sleek adolescent as summer progressed. The town was divided over the rights of that little family. It was one of those cocktail-party subjects to be avoided, along with religion and politics. The pro-goose and antigoose factions made no secret of their dismay at the unreasoned folly of the opposing side. "Next year they will be back, and they'll bring their friends. That baby will grow up and bring his mate. Before you know it, you won't want your children playing on the beach. Before you know it, we'll look just like Kelly Drive." This reference to Philadelphia draws immediate recognition in a town whose summer population comes mainly from that area. I'm amused by all the fuss. It is usually New Yorkers who inspire this kind of concern. Osprey Lakes is certain we will become commercialized just like the Poconos as soon as we are discovered by those in Manhattan. But that year, at least in the eyes of some, those three geese were seen to be as potentially threatening as an invasion from the Big Apple.

Unfortunately, one day when Chuckles and I sought solitude away from the summer crowd's enthusiasm for the Laurel Path, we dove right into the controversy over the three Canadians. We live quite close to the Outlet Pond and must pass it on our way to the relative seclusion of the railroad bed. A few cars were parked in the Outlet Pond parking lot, and one woman was scattering bread crumbs to the geese as they waddled about on the bank. As soon as the goose family saw Chuckles coming, they set up an ungodly squawking and hollering. Even the baby managed a teenager's cracked-voice rendition of his parents' alarm. Chuckles took it as a call to action and charged after them. They hit the water running, and he splashed smartly in after them, swimming as fast as he could in their direction. Since the youngster could not yet fly, he merely flapped his wings madly over the surface of the water. The parents flapped beside him but refused to go airborne without their son.

Dog owners make excuses for wayward charges as easily as do parents, and I am no exception. Chuckles is a wimp. As soon as the geese stopped swimming and turned to face him, he gave up and paddled back to shore. I knew he wouldn't hurt the geese. This is the same dog who spit a nestful of live baby rabbits gently into my hand. This is the same dog who gambols like a puppy, wagging his tail and laughing when he chases the occasional shrew trapped momentarily on the crusted surface of the snow. Chuckles seems to want to play with his quarry. Killing it appears to be the last thing in his mind. Still, he is a clumsy Lenny of a dog, and it's true I can't guarantee that harm won't someday come to one of his "playmates." I suppose I should have stopped him from chasing the geese, but his entry into the water was so filled with joy and my vision of the outcome was so benign, I couldn't bring myself to take charge. The various lookers-on had no such problem.

"Dogs ought to be on leads!"

What saved me on that day was the presence of more than one party witnessing the chase. The debate quickly shifted from me and my dog to the pro-goose/antigoose controversy.

"You should hope to heaven that dog tells those geese to nest somewhere else next year," rejoined one woman who will ever have a special place in my unrepentant heart.

"All wild creatures need protecting."

"Did I see you feeding those geese? That's all they need, just a little encouragement and you'll turn them into permanent panhandlers. Come fall and they won't even fly south," our defender continued.

"I just wanted them to get close enough so I could take a picture."

Chuckles and I didn't wait to see how the debate turned out. We made our exit with me muttering, "He wouldn't chase them if they didn't honk."

A lot happens in the natural world in March, but socially the town is quiet. Gossip fills the void. Being relative newcomers, we are at the bottom of the gossip chain. Which means that by the time the stories make their way down to us, they have been sufficiently embellished that they really are worth repeating. The only trouble is there is no one to tell who hasn't already heard the yarn. One of my favorite March tales is of the holdup attempt at the Barn restaurant (read bar). Now, this is more than the story of a robbery. It is the story of a romance. It's a classic fable of a longtime couple who had gone their separate ways only to be reunited by an act of bravery.

The Barn is the favorite watering hole of those who have called Osprey Lakes home for generations. Darlene Lopez and Ronnie Houst had been a couple of such long standing that their breakup came as a shock to the whole town. But so deeply ingrained were their patterns of togetherness that no one, not even Darlene and Ronnie, seemed to find it odd that they continued to go to the same places at the same time. On the night in question, they were sitting side by side, but definitely not together, on their accustomed barstools. By early evening, the bar had filled with the usual crowd. Since the late-winter months can be a slow time in the trades that keep local folk employed, some of the regulars had already moved past mere unwinding. Kay Wilson, who is Houst-connected, was doing one of her relatives a favor by filling in as bartender that night. Unraveling the web of Sullivan County degrees of relatedness could keep an anthropologist with a specialty in kinship busy for years. The best advice to a newcomer is, pass on no local gossip locally. Everyone is related to everyone else by marriage, birth, or affection.

Suddenly, someone wearing a ski mask and waving a gun burst through the door. He ran over to the bar and pointed the gun at Kay, demanding that she empty the cash register. She, thinking the masked man was one of her relatives playing a prank on her, began to laugh. The gunman was momentarily nonplussed, but soon came up with a counterplan and began working his way down the lineup at the bar, demanding cash from each in turn. However, the regulars at the Barn run a tab, and no one had any cash to give him. By the time he got to Darlene, his patience and his temper had worn thin. He pointed the gun directly at her temple: "Somebody'd better pay up, or I'll blow her head off."

Ronnie, disgusted with the display of incompetence, bellowed angrily, "Shoot her or get the fuck out!"

The would-be robber had had enough. He turned and ran out the door a whole lot faster than he had run in. He was never found, but it can only be assumed that he headed back to Philadelphia where people at least know how to behave during a stickup.

The story isn't quite over. The state police cross-examined the witnesses one by one in the back room, but couldn't come up with any two descriptions that bore any resemblance whatsoever to each other. Ronnie was interviewed on the Wilkes-Barre television nightly news and quickly became a local celebrity. You can guess the ending. Heroism proved an irresistible aphrodisiac, and true love and harmony returned to the mountain. March is always an interesting month in Osprey Lakes.

My great-aunt Bay was the undisputed matriarch of our family. Although she'd never married, she'd had a hand (a firm hand) in raising my mother and her brothers. Back in the politically incorrect 1940s, she was described by everyone who knew her as an old-maid schoolteacher. Most of the residents of Roxborough had passed through her classroom, and they all stood up straighter when they saw Miss Carberry walking down the street. To my knowledge, I'm the only person who ever crossed Bay. I was four at the time. The story of my encounter quickly moved into family legend. Perhaps the most remarkable thing about it is that Bay herself not only backed down in the face of my challenge, but found the story amusing enough to repeat. The arena for our battle was the crown jewel in Bay's scrubbed and gleaming household, the Sunday stairs. There was another flight that led from the kitchen to the upper floors, and those were the stairs that everyone was required to use. Except on Sunday. On Sunday, passage was permitted on the waxed and polished perfection of the front staircase. On the day in question, Bay was watching me while my mother took my sisters to the dentist. Because I was a shy child, Bay was unacquainted with the ferocious rage all too familiar to my immediate family members. I can't remember what she did or said that day to push me into an emotional corner. But I do remember my response. I skittered across her front parlor and hopped up onto the bottom step of the forbidden stairway. Defiantly locking eyes with her, I extended one leg and strategically poised the sharp edge of the heel of my brown, laced oxford on the waxed surface. Rigid with fear and fury, I stopped her advance toward me with the threat "I'll scratch your Sunday stairs!"

Chapter 12

April

When I was first diagnosed with cancer, I reassured all my Carberry relatives by telling them, "Don't worry. I'm going to scratch this cancer's Sunday stairs." They believed me, more, I think, than I believed myself. Family members know me for my fierce determination. I alone am familiar with the fear that inspires it. What am I to make now of this apparent good health? Can it be true? Have I really stopped this disease as surely as I stopped Aunt Bay? My good health has a fragile, tentative feel to it. Is it really okay to relax, unclench my fists, just get on with my life?

April makes it easy to believe. Sweet, soft April stirs and lifts, relaxing everything. Even the lake is suddenly alive once more. The lake usually thaws in March, but this year the ice held on. It wasn't until last week that three days of wind shattered the frozen surface into millions of little shards that pushed against the shore with a musical tinkling incomparable to anything else. Water chimes. When Gene and I walked Chuckles, we walked without speaking, so reluctant were we to miss even an instant of this glorious symphony of spring.

The music doesn't happen every year. Sometimes a week of sodden rain just slowly melts the ice. Sometimes it is a combination of rain and fog. And sometimes it is a series of sunny, still days that form spreading pools of water on the surface until gradually the whole lake is open water. I prefer the drama of wind and ice chimes. But regardless of how the lake thaws, one thing astonishes me every year: the sudden return of movement to a previously frozen world. The lake is alive! The surface dances and sparkles. I can't take my eyes off it. Tiny waves and ripples reach from shore to shore, reflecting fluid light. All the energy that had been locked in by rigid cold is joyously released.

March and April are waterfowl migration months. We get Canadian geese whether the lake has thawed or not. But not until there is open water does the real spectacle begin. Once the lake thaws, I don't leave the house without my binoculars and bird book. I was not a "birder" until we moved to Osprey Lakes. Even now, I'm not good with songbirds. They flit about too fast. Only those that frequent my feeder are reliably identified. But waterfowl are a novice's delight. They sit still on an open body of water allowing time to study every detail, check the book, and then return to the same bird for more study. There are no branches or leaves in the way. I don't have to rely on flight patterns and song for clues. They are simply there, sitting ducks, so to speak.

There is a further attraction to waterfowl migrations, the sheer dramatic unpredictability of the whole affair. Most of the geese and ducks we see are transients, on their way to somewhere else. So each one has a sense of the miraculous about it. The half dozen goldeneyes rapidly whistling just above the surface of the lake may be gone by the time we take our afternoon walk. I might not see them again this season or for several seasons to come. Except for Canada geese and loons, which have reliably returned every spring and fall since we have lived here, the waterfowl are random tourists. We must be located just to one side of the usual flyway. It takes wind or fog, some gift of weather, to bring them to us. Some years Canada geese, loons, and an occasional mallard constitute the entire spring or fall migration. But I can tell already that this April of fickle weather patterns and shifting winds is going to be a glorious one for waterbirds.

One day last week, there was a steady, hard north wind. The lake was covered with so many species of ducks I couldn't count them all. Fred even saw a snow goose flying in formation with a bunch of Canadas, her white body and half-black wings a standout next to her darker companions. When we first moved up here, five snow geese and two whistling swans swooped down and stayed with us for most of one day. That was a rare enough occurrence that even people who don't usually get excited about ducks on the lake made a special trip down to the beach just to catch a glimpse of them.

Last weekend's assortment contained nothing so dramatic as swans, but there was enough activity that our hour-long dog walk stretched to two as Gene and I handed binoculars and bird books back and forth debating and naming. It was the first time I had ever seen, or at least the first time I had accurately identified, ring-necked ducks and lesser scaups on our lake. And at least fifty old-squaws bobbed about swimming and diving, their needle-like tail feathers and flashy black-and-white patterns making identification easy but, nonetheless, exciting. In addition to those, buffleheads, horned grebes, hooded mergansers, red-breasted mergansers, and the uncommonly beautiful common mergansers all delighted us with a visit of several days. The wind was cold enough to hold them here and strong enough to blow them close to the southwestern shore where we could get a good look.

Yesterday I spotted a small flock of maybe fourteen or fifteen wood ducks on the lake. Once again, it was a first-time sighting for me. They are elusive, agile swimmers, and when they take flight, it is rapid. I happen to think a male wood duck is the most beautiful of birds. Stunning as photographs of wood ducks are, nothing comes close to the splendor of this creature seen in full feather. Both the male and female have crested heads, but his is etched in dark, iridescent stripes alternating with white. His eye and beak are bright red. A vertical band of white separates his ruddy breast from buff sides and a back that reflects green, purple, and blue. Wild to share my sighting with someone, I called Craig as soon as I got home. He had seen wood ducks of his own, but because the pair that he had spotted were on the Outlet Pond, they were available for closer study.

I took the binoculars down to the shore closest to the Conservancy cabin and waited. There was movement in the reeds under the blueberry bushes on the northern banks. This is a wonderful spot for wood ducks. There are rotting logs at the edge of the water and dead trees not far from shore. Wood ducks nest in trees. Although I wished that they would raise their young here, I knew better. We have too much summertime activity for them to be willing to build their nests in so public a spot. The sun was at a low angle, and every rich color of the male was spotlighted as he drifted into my lens. For once I got to enjoy the markings on both the male and the female for almost as long as I wanted. When they finally disappeared into the shallow water behind the bleached gold of the reeds, I turned my sights to other things. Another pair of ducks was on the pond, and these were as plain as the wood ducks were spectacular.

This dowdy duo had me stumped. I looked at every illustration in two different bird books and couldn't find anything that looked exactly like the two that calmly paddled about in front of me. They acted like a bonded pair, and so I assumed, possibly falsely, that they were a male and female. They were a dull gray or blackish brown, no distinctive color markings at all. Not even the sun could bring any reflected beauty to their feathers. One of them, but not the other, seemed to have pale cheek patches. However, it was hard to tell. Sometimes they tucked their heads under their wings and just drifted with the current. They were divers, and I thought perhaps their very wetness was hiding some identifying mark. So fascinated was I by their inscrutability, that even when the wood ducks reappeared, I was unable to turn my lens away from that which I could not know. Gathering darkness finally drove me back to the house, where I sat and recorded the day's sightings. The last entry read, "April 8, 1993, two ugly?"

When Gene drove in from Philly, he promised we would figure it out by morning. And not long after sunrise, we were dutifully out there. We have several candidates but still can't be sure. Craig is likewise stumped, but he tells me that when he takes Erin and Kyle to the pond fishing tonight, he will come up with an answer. I can feel myself beginning to love this pair. They seem happy in our waters. The fishing must be good. In fact, it is their sweeping dives that have made Craig get the itch to fish himself. There is a contentment about them, a cozy companionship. When you see one, you see the other. Even their dives are synchronized. I begin to regret calling them ugly. How horrible to base my entire assessment on the dullness of their feathers. Surely this devotion, surely this joy in April and each other, count for something.

It's late afternoon. I know by the tone of Chuckles' bark that Craig's truck has pulled up in front of our house. I hear Gene asking what's wrong, and by the time I get to the door, Craig's sad face telegraphs fear through me. "Erin? Kyle?" is all I can manage in anguished inquiry.

He shakes his head. "They're fine. It's the ducks—one of the ducks was killed. I have it in the truck."

The story is a sad one. A power line runs parallel to the bridge that separates the lake from the Outlet Pond. A couple of years ago someone fishing from the bridge tangled his line around the electric wires. I've hated the way that line and bobber dangle in front of what would otherwise be a clear view of the pond, but the thought of standing with my feet in water while pulling at a length of fishing line attached to a source of power stopped me from ever doing anything about it. Now I rue my inaction.

Craig and the kids were standing on the east shore of the pond. The first time he cast, he startled our anonymous pair, and they took flight. One of the ducks hit the nearly invisible line hanging from the electric wires and, taking the line down with her, fell to the surface of the lake, dead. I follow Craig out to his truck. He lifts her so tenderly. Her body is still soft. He moves one hand under her head to support the flopping neck. She is drab no more. Two slashes of bright crimson, one between her eyes and another across her breast, accent the dull gray feathers. Craig, Gene, and I study her sadly. Then Gene says, "We've got her here. We might as well." Craig has a bird book in his glove compartment. We turn the pages. No problem here. Surf Scoter. We all agree.

After I return to the house, I drag out my notebook, erase *ugly ?* from last night's entry and write in *Surf Scoter*. I look at what I've done and realize something is still not right. Sadly, sadly, I erase *two* and pencil in the up-to-date information. *One Surf Scoter*. I think of that other one, out there alone on the darkening water, and desperately hope that by tomorrow morning he has flown. I don't want to see the pattern of his movement through the water, solitary ripples where once there were overlapping circles. Death is a problem for the living, not the dying, or at least not for the already dead. But how can I be certain even of this?

My mother died when she was eighty. Her death was no surprise. She had endured years of severe emphysema with the same stoicism that she suffered a life whose gifts of joy were hard won from a thirty-year history of mental illness. This delusional depression was misdiagnosed as schizophrenia, and the horror of the drugs we forced on her caused damage more grave than the disease they mistakenly sought to cure. Only in her eightieth year did lithium restore balance and give her back her own personality.

Even in its best times, my mother's life was hard, almost from the beginning. *Her* mother had died when Mother was very young. A handsome, charming but hot-tempered father used Mother as a pawn in fights with various relatives, and she was pulled from one home to another whenever he had one of his frequent blow-ups. At age seven, she was largely responsible for her two younger brothers. And when she grew up and married, her husband, my father, was again a charming, handsome ladies' man who had too many loud opinions, too forcefully held. There was more to Mother than life allowed her to express. More fury and more happiness. Only in that last year of her life did she begin to share unadorned vignettes from her childhood: "When I was twelve, Bay said that we were getting too old to get Christmas presents, and there would be none that year. But, of course, when Christmas came, I was the only one who didn't get any presents."

Of course. I remember taking her to the doctor just a few months before she died. She was fiercely modest and always insisted that I accompany her into the examining room. Dr. Genetti greeted her warmly. People loved my mother. I think they sensed the toughness and the humor behind her speak-only-when-spoken-to reticence. He looked at her anxiously and then inquired as to the state of her health. "How are you doing, Hazel?"

"Fine, thank you. How are you?"

"You seem to be breathing pretty heavily."

"Oh, that doesn't mean anything. I always breathe like that."

Dr. Genetti listened to her heart, took her blood pressure, peered into her mouth with a tongue depressor and flashlight. He then told her he wanted to do a breast exam and began listing statistics on the incidence of cancer in the elderly. Mother refused. Dr. Genetti turned to me for support, and Mother interrupted his campaign. "I have to die of something. It might as well be of that." There was no breast exam done on that day or on any other day in her all too short future. Mother seemed to have a comfortable acceptance of death, certainly a more realistic one than that evidenced by most of the medical profession.

So a dream I had a few months after her death surprises me. Here I anticipate all the protests of the psychiatric profession, that wonderful bunch who subjected her to thirty years of torture. I *know* that my dreams reveal my psyche, not my mother's. I know equally that this was a dream, pure and simple, no visitation from some ghostly realm. Still, having said all that, her presence was so real and our exchange so in keeping with the nature of her living conversations that the words do seem to be hers and not my own. In the dream, I am standing in an apartment that is now my father's alone. There are bay windows. Light is refracted through leaded glass. Suddenly, Mother is there, just surveying the room with a quizzical look on her face. She walks over and opens the closet door, runs her left hand critically over my father's suits hanging on racks that have an unnatural amount of space. "Why, he's taken all my clothes out of the closet," she says in a voice tinged with quiet indignation. There is also a hint of exasperation at the presumptive folly by which she knew this man.

It's hard for me to admit it now, but when I was a child, I played the role of Daddy's defender. In the dream I fall back into the old position, trying to make some excuse for what he has done, to offer some explanation that will color the action and make it all okay. I don't know how to begin to tell her that she doesn't live here anymore. I walk over to her and find my most gentle voice. I lovingly put one arm around her shoulder. "Mother," I quietly tell her, "you died. You are dead."

My mother is a small woman. Old age and ill health have made her even smaller and more frail. Now she pulls herself up and says with all the sad dignity she can muster, "Yes, I know that." But her face belies her words. There is so much regret there. I awake, hating to awaken, wanting the dream back in all its sad, unspoken longing, wanting my mother back, and her life back, but not the one she had. I want the life that was taken from her. I want her to have joy.

What is this thing called death? All around me this sweet April I see life. By the middle of the month, the last traces of snow are gone. Not even in the sheltered, shadowed cliffs and caves does any trace remain. Spring comes at me in a rush. The green shoots of the bulbs Dee and I fought into the rocky ground are pushing forth with near-visible speed, the whole world recorded in the time-lapse photography of the human eye. There are not yet leaves on any trees, but in one warm day the Tartarian honeysuckle, scrub brush, near-weed, will be transformed. Unclothed, its dry branches lack any pleasing symmetry, but give it twelve hours of sun and its brand-new green leaves will validate the season. I saw my first spring beauties, pale pink and white, in the woods beside the airport. The roadsides are yellow with Coltsfoot, mistaken for dandelion by most who see it blooming there.

The ospreys are back. Now when Chuckles and I take our afternoon walk, they come calling out of the tops of ancient, wind-sculpted pines near the beach. I stand on the dock and watch their majesty in stunned amazement. What is this thing called death? Yesterday one circled the lake, poised and gliding, flapping those arching wings just enough to give direction to his flight or hold himself briefly suspended. And then, suddenly, down he dropped, diving, splashing, reaching deep below the surface; he dove, then struggled to come back up, a gravity-defying thrust of wings, thrashing, pushing against the water with labored strength. When he at last lifted free and was airborne, he clasped a shining, dripping fish in his talons. What is this thing called death? I am at once osprey and trout, the living and the dying, the fed and fed-upon. I can't separate the two, or myself from either.

Life is the defining characteristic of this world, the world we know. And every form of life we see is nourished only by the death of something else. My spring beauties bloom in decaying leaves. The osprey must have his trout, and I my rice, broccoli, and beans. I can't make the Buddhist's distinction between sentient and insentient life. All life is holy, the tree no less so than the owl on its branch. Lacking the osprey's honest confrontation with what and who I am, I remove myself from the moment of death that brings broiled haddock to my plate. Although I hate the thought of a deer crumpling inert, pierced through by a rifle shell, I can't condemn the hunter who carries home his venison. The hunter does his own killing. I hire others to do mine for me. I live only when something else dies. We all live only through the death of something else. What is this thing called death? It is so much a part of life, so much the source of life, that it can only be called the precursor of life. It is not an end but a beginning.

What happens when we die? I think of this as I walk the perimeter of the airport, caught up in the glorious unfolding of this new season. I stoop gently to cup the first trout lily, its clear yellow flower vibrant above the speckled green leaves that inspire its name. Nearby, mayapples, their umbrella-shaped leaves still folded into tiny spears, heave through the earth. The sun is sinking. The wide expanse of the mountaintop open space stretches my soul from horizon to horizon. The sweet transport of this moment between the seasons is so filled with joy. Surely the moment of death must be the same. The magic and the mystery are all captured there in the brief pulse between what was and what will be.

I don't see death as winter coming on. Winter is a frozen, rigid, waiting time. Death is a bursting forth, a shedding of dry cocoons, a great leap forward into something less confining. I *want* death to take my boundaries, dissolve my ego, set me free to soar and glide.

A friend once asked if I wanted to be cremated or buried in the more conventional style and was surprised at my choice of cremation. She was curious as to the reasons. My answer was flippant: "I don't find rotting flesh very attractive." But when I thought about it later, I knew I hadn't told the truth. It is a lack of rotting flesh that is unnatural and abhorrent. I don't want to be embalmed in some futile and misguided attempt to halt the march of time. I don't want a moisture-proof, high-tech casket designed to keep the elements out. I want to let the elements in. Allow nothing to stand between me and the natural world and my place in it. Bring on the worms and let that which was my body give rise to something green and growing. I prefer cremation to the extended state of inanimation that marks modern burial practices. I suspect that the same regulations that dictate the interment of embalmed bodies govern as well the disposal of cremated remains. However, I also suspect that those laws are easier to break when one is dealing with a small container of ash and charred bone, everything purified by heat and flame.

On the brief drive back from the airport, Chuckles and I stop to check the status of the leeks. Ingrid has called this morning. She and friends are coming up for the annual ham and leek dinner at the Endless Winds Fire Hall in Shunk. This year it's scheduled for the last weekend of the month, and Ing and I are both worried that due to the catch-up haste with which spring is exploding, our local ramps will be past their prime. Chuckles, never one to question good fortune, leaps joyously from the car as if this extra stop were a regular part of our afternoons. He bounces through the woods in the stiff-legged, gazellelike leaps he uses to raise himself above the ground cover for a clear view of any creatures who might be lurking there. I laugh and call after him, "Imaginary squirrels, old boy!" I can see nothing and turn my attention from him to the forest floor.

Everywhere, as far as I can see, smooth new-green leaves herald an abundant harvest in our secret gathering ground. Mixed all through the onion-

scented leeks are the showy white blossoms of bloodroot. Two of my favorite things intermingled in such a glorious display. The bloodroot is just
starting to bloom. Its pale green, lobed leaves are still cupped, barely unfolding, at the base of the slender stalk. My intention had been to dig a few
leeks, push the rich black humus off with my thumb, and sit here munching
away. There is no one at home to take offense at my reeking, telltale breath,
but once here, I cannot do it. It is not wise to eat leeks alone, not unless one
is certain one wishes to remain truly alone. But there is more to it than that.
I am surrounded by such harmonious perfection that I can't bring myself to
rearrange one leaf.

Despite their reputation as savage onions, leeks are actually a member of
the lily family. However, they won't bloom with a spokelike umbel of white
flowers until after the leaves have withered. For now, they look like lilies of
the valley minus the little bells that characterize that more familiar species.
I happily conclude that the volunteer firemen in Shunk know their leeks, and
I anticipate informing Ingrid that all appears to be right on schedule.

Even as a child, I loved bloodroot as much for its name as for the tender
beauty of its white, waxen blossoms, its gold-dusted stamens. Purity. Sim-
plicity. Truth. When picked, its slender stem stains the fingers orange. Something deeply elemental here, something mythical, beyond logic. I try to
articulate now what my childhood self had understood without recourse to
words. Bloodroot heralds the fusion between rooted plant and beating heart,
marks the place where life meets life. I kneel over one plant, inhaling deeply.
It has no hint of fragrance strong enough to cancel out its more assertive leek
neighbors, but the movement, the deep intake of breath, the rush of blood
to my head tosses and catches me in that sweet tumbled cycle of impermanence and renewal through which I know the gods.

Chuckles barks sharply, pulling me back to more practical issues. He is
face-to-face with a large porcupine. Chuckles has met a porcupine once before. He made the mistake of trying to pick that one up and suffered all the
subsequent anguish that comes of such introductions rudely undertaken.
This evening he is offering a more mannerly and cautious invitation to play.
Forelegs flat on the ground, rump elevated and anchor to a madly wagging
plume of tail, he tosses his head back and forth in a coaxing manner. "Chuckles!" I scream. "Chuckles. No! Down. Come!" In my panic, I throw every
command he ever has been taught into a jumbled mélange of contradicting

orders. Luckily for us both, and for the porcupine as well I suppose, Chuckles responds to my terror and not my words. Looking crestfallen, he slinks back to me, belly to the ground in anticipation of some punishment. Instead, I shower him with hugs, kisses, pats, praise, and good-boys. Flooded with relief, I watch the porcupine turn and slowly waddle off. He seems quite unconcerned. If there is terror in his heart, he doesn't let it show. Only when the porcupine is safely up the nearest tree do I release my hold on Chuckles.

I love the measured ritual of my days. In April I fall asleep to the sound of spring peepers, awake to birds. Before I run, I feed Chuckles and Spike. They share in my daybreak tribute to the healing power of herbs. As I boil my tea, dark bitter mix of dandelion and burdock root, red clover, ginseng, slippery elm, pau d'arco, and sheep sorrel, I almost chant the words. There is some magic in those names, suma, astralagus, rhubarb. The cat and the dog don't drink the tea. I give them tablets of brewer's yeast and garlic instead, but we all take pollen products, sweet gifts of the hive, the bee, the natural world. I crave solitude the first waking hour of every day. Those who love me know to stay in their beds until I have worked my way through the due order of this liturgy. It is my daily celebration of health, of continuity, of life.

Now that I am stronger, I write three to five hours a day, five days a week. *Out of England* has taken me much longer to complete than I had anticipated. When I was bargaining for time with my doctors, afraid to ask for more than they could safely promise, I claimed it would be finished in six months, then begged for a year. Now, almost twelve months later, I continue to plod away. I suspect that many of the chapters written while in the throes of chemotherapy will need to be rewritten, but I struggle to set judgment aside and simply lose myself in the process. It is a fight each morning. I resist, make excuses, circle the typewriter suspiciously, but when I finally break through the barrier of that first half hour, the rest is effortless. The discipline of place and time, the rites of tea and chewing gum, and sharpened pencils override the hopeless sense of inadequacy to the task at hand. Soon one word follows another, each dictated by the one before it, with no apparent input of my own. It's as if it all belongs to someone else. I am divorced from the product, divorced from everything but the joy of creation flowing through me. *Out of England* was to be the tool with which I would remake the world into a more just place. I wonder now if anyone will ever read it, or if it has simply been the tool with which I have remade myself.

I have come full circle. It is spring again, and I'm still here. Willis is back on the mountain. I hadn't seen him since he brought the last load of wood in late November. He and the great blue herons arrive at about the same time. The herons gather fish, and Willis moves across the yards bundling the dead branches and sticks brought down by winter storms. Soon the music of his mower will fill the air. And soon the summer people will be back, and his battles with those who sleep too late will begin once more. People tell me the winter has been hard on Willis, that he is more stooped than before, but I don't see it. He comes to visit me in the late afternoon. He has a working person's respect for the hours I reserve for writing. I always offer Willis tea, but only once has he accepted. True to form, today he shakes his head in polite refusal. "No, no. Don't have time for that. I just came by to see how you're doing."

"Willis," I happily tell him, "I'm fine, just absolutely fine."

He looks at me quizzically. "That old cancer gone?"

"Gone without a trace. They did blood tests, they did CAT scans, gone without a trace."

"Well, I'll be." He shakes his head in smiling disbelief. "Well now, that's real good. That sure is real good news."

We catch up on a winter's worth of talk. The concrete things, wildlife sightings, family, and weather. Willis has a new remedy for arthritis. "You know that stuff they use to loosen bolts, WD-40? Well, you spray just a bit of that on your knees, then rub it in. You ought to see me. I can go right up and down them cellar steps. It sure does seem to make a difference. But, be careful," he tells me. "Don't use too much. You know it will take a bolt right off." He laughs with the old teasing twinkle. "I wouldn't want you to use too much."

I promise I'll run down to Dave's and Diane's Hardware and get a can, which I will use cautiously. I have a vague image of my lower leg suddenly disconnecting from the knee. Before Willis leaves, I hand him a small bottle of my own favorite herbal capsules, but the offering seems tame and undramatic next to WD-40. I watch as he walks slowly back to his truck. He is so dear, so familiar, so much a part of all the reasons why I can't trade this life for the unknown, no matter how potentially glorious.

It's perfect weather for the ham and leek supper. Ingrid, John, and Ingrid's friend Sarah are astonished that we still don't have any leaves on the trees. They have come in from Philadelphia where spring is already moving on toward summer. A gang of us are going to eat the meal prepared by Shunk's volunteer firemen and their wives. Craig and Dee and the kids, our trio of urban types, assorted friends from Osprey Lakes, and Gene and me. The only torture is that we can't all fit in one vehicle, and I will be forced to imagine conversations I can't hear. I know Ing and Craig are laughing in the car ahead of us. The love between this brother and sister is so strong, despite the difference in their lifestyles. My country mouse, my city mouse.

The drive to Shunk is incredibly beautiful. The colors of early spring are even more varied than those of fall, but the effect is subtle, the contrast muted. The Endless Mountains are appropriately named. One gently rounded peak rolls into the other. High farmland pastures are carved out of hills and forest, their shape dictated by geographic contour in a flowing harmony. The maple trees are all in bloom, russet, dusky rose, bronze, and transparent gold. Robert Frost claimed

> Nature's first green is gold,
> Her hardest hue to hold.

Each year, in April, I recite his words. My former melancholy self found truth, believed the rest of the poem and knew catharsis in the lines

> Her early leaf's a flower;
> But only so an hour.
> Then leaf subsides to leaf.
> So Eden sank to grief,
> So dawn goes down to day.
> Nothing gold can stay.

I used to subscribe to that opinion. I still know that spring is fleeting. The moments move so fast that, turn away for just an instant and you will have missed it. But the gold does stay. I understand that now. It merely transmutes into an overlay of other shades and colors. It is always there, that nub of first life, under everything, waiting for the wheel to turn, waiting for another season, another year, another life risen out of the old.

If you arrive late at a community supper in Sullivan County, the food may be all gone. We never take a chance in Shunk, are always there well before six. A good thing, because already the line stretches all the way down along the side of the fire hall and into the back parking lot. It is a laughing, salivating crowd. The aromas emanating from the building leave no doubt that leeks are on the menu, and the time passes quickly with tales of former suppers, the numbers of bushels consumed, and favorite leek moments. The small, gray-haired woman in front of us remembers her first year of teaching in a rural county school.

"It was a one-room schoolhouse. I'd been there since September. Well, this was April and the superintendent was coming in somewhere from all the other way down in the county to observe me teach. Oh, but I was scared. Well, the day he finally came turned out to be the day the children decided the leeks were ready to gather. Of course, I didn't know just which day he was going to come. By the time those youngsters got to the schoolhouse, they'd been all through the woods, digging and eating leeks. Oh my, but they did smell! I could hardly stand it, but they told me to eat a few myself and then I wouldn't notice. So I did. I'd never had a leek before and I didn't like them much, but the trick worked, and I couldn't smell anything at all. Well, wouldn't you know it, I'd no sooner than turned around when in came the superintendent. I could see him sniffing, so I had the children open up all the windows, and I thought it worked because it seemed okay to me." She pauses here to laugh, the memory still so fresh. "I must have been wrong because he only stayed fifteen minutes or so. All that long drive and he only stayed fifteen minutes. I've liked leeks ever since!"

It's starting to rain, and we all press in close under the eaves. Soon the big garage doors roll open and several apron-clad ladies urge us to come and stand in among the fire trucks. The fire trucks and the pies! Tables are set up all along one wall and on them must be at least one hundred pies. Only little Kyle is more enchanted with the fire trucks than with the desserts. The rest of us stand in front of those tables debating the merits of chocolate cream versus strawberry rhubarb, apple as opposed to cherry. The lemon meringue glistens with tiny beads of moisture on its stiff and curling peaks. We observe the intricacies of crust design. The crimped edges come in as many forms as the hands that shaped them. We make a game of trying to assign pies according to the signature imprint of the various women of this community.

People are here to eat. The main hall is lined with rows of long, folding tables, and every seat is filled with laughing, chewing people. As they return to load their plates with second and third helpings, those in process call encouragement to those of us still in line. They promise not to eat it all, and we believe them. As fast as one serving platter is emptied, steaming replacements arrive. There appears to be a limitless supply of food, but experience has taught me that it will all be gone before dark. Six dollars apiece for adults; children six through twelve are three dollars; and Erin and Kyle, given that they are both under six, are free. Big families with large broods take advantage of this night. You would be amazed how much a child under six can eat at a ham and leek dinner. The pricing reflects the inclusive nature of the community, the value placed on children far more than any calculations of bottom line.

At last we grab empty plates and begin loading up. Ham and mashed potatoes running with gravy, leeks simmered in the cooking juices of the ham, crusty baked beans, corn, rolls, Jell-O salad, and coleslaw, homemade pies, coffee, and punch. The menu never varies. By the time we reach the end of the table, not one of us has the smallest fraction of plate showing through our mounds of food. We compare degrees of gluttony, admire artful banking techniques, and wonder which of us will be the first to return to line. The tables are set with all manner of condiments, but the crowning glory is dish after dish of raw leeks. They gleam white as polished ivory. There is a bowl within arm's reach of everyone. As fast as we clean one bowl out, the smiling women who circulate through the room are there to fill it up again. The bulb of a raw leek bites back, but the green leaves are an offsetting blend reminiscent of woods and dandelion.

At our urging, Kyle gamely tries a raw leek. The whole table laughs at his resultant expression, and thus encouraged he turns his attention to the comedic properties of leeks. We are treated to walrus fangs, elephant trunks, leeks behind the ears, and unicornlike horns. At this stage of his life, leeks are more fun to play with than to eat. At last, bored with the game, he works his way through a second mound of mashed potatoes. We've lost count of how much ham and Jell-O salad he has consumed. Erin is securely jammed in between her aunt Ingrid and Sarah. Enchanted by this glamorous aunt and her friend, Erin mimics every gesture that they make. She will eat whatever Aunt Ingrid is eating. My plate is empty. I haven't consumed this much at one sitting since the last ham and leek dinner I was able to attend two years ago.

I'm counting my blessings. All these happy faces: friends, family, strangers, seated at the table sharing in our laughter. Gene catches my eye from across the table. We smile and both fill up with tears. I look at our grandchildren, carried by love, nurtured by parents whose devotion to each other and them is plain to anyone fortunate enough to witness the cherishing acceptance with which they speak and touch. What must it be like to be so loved? I wonder. The chain of depression that has linked the generations of my family seems finally broken. The ring of love extends beyond the little family before me, and into the community, one bright circle after another. Erin and Kyle know Frank, the postmaster and deputy game warden; J.R., who owns the local convenience store; Enza, the tax collector; Jay, who dips cones at the Sweet Shop; Frank Shoemaker, who plows our roads, picks up our trash, and keeps all things in working order; Pam, the borough secretary and Girl Scout leader; Shelly, baby-sitter, postal clerk, waitress; Chet, schoolbus driver and mechanic who fixes Baboo's funny little car; Bea, the poet who signs her book with special verses just for them; Jerry, the contractor whose claim to fame for Kyle and Erin is his way with backhoes; Jimmy, housepainter, pilot of the *Hardly Able*, keeper of all the boats; one hundred and twenty-three year-round residents love and are loved by these two lucky little people. I watch them wave and call hello to latecomers just arriving. Erin and Kyle do not find it strange that their community is always so reliably there. This bond is all they know.

I go with Ingrid and Erin, my two girls, to decide on dessert. Our preliminary scouting has been no help at all. "Which would you have," I ask the woman serving up the slices, "the chocolate cream or the strawberry rhubarb?"

"Why don't you just take one of each?"

Erin is enchanted with this option. She looks up at her aunt Ingrid in grinning disbelief. "Can I?"

"Are you hungry enough to eat two pieces?" Ingrid asks cautiously.

Erin nods and Ing tells her, "Then go for it, girl!"

There is something in the tilt of Erin's head, some shadow that moves across her cheek, the half-smile, the half-light, some motion there that blurs my eyes and carries me to old photographs of my mother as a child. For just one fleeting heartbeat, it is my mother captured there before me in the joy of a life overflowing with a happy surfeit of choices. I bend to kiss the top of Erin's head. I run my hand behind her ear. She moves away from me, and I stand frozen in that crowded room and watch my daughter guide my grand-daughter, a piece of pie in each hand, back to our table. It takes me a little while to catch my breath. How can one person hold so much happiness as is mine? This leek-filled rite of spring is heady stuff. Impermanence. Renewal. Impermanence. Renewal. The pulse of life celebrates all our sorrows and our joys. It echoes and transcends the beating heart. Everything is measured there in its steady rhythm, its steady, constant, and enduring rhythm.